Praise for *Pandemics and Politics*:

"A fascinating and moving story of a lifetime dedicated to science and global health. Max Essex provides us with a close-up view of the evolution over half a century in both attitudes and capacities in the battle against pandemic disease. His is at once an uplifting chronicle of progress and a frustrating record of how we have so often created obstacles to our own success."

Drew Faust, Author of *This Republic of Suffering* and President Emerita, Harvard University

"Max Essex spent five decades sleuthing the mysteries of how viruses cause diseases. His work on African AIDS at Botswana Harvard helped to discover how to prevent infant infections, a high-water mark both for American humanism and for the scientific power of international collaboration. The book offers essential lessons for those who will one day rebuild America's leadership in global health – foremost, that politics has the power to destroy science."

Elizabeth Finkel, Award-winning Journalist and Author of *Prove It*

"Max Essex's lifetime of research – from his early work on feline retroviruses, which helped convince me that a human retrovirus might cause AIDS, to developing strategies that reduced the devastation of AIDS in Africa – is science at its finest. This book is both a testament to the best of medical research and a powerful lesson in how the destructive forces of denialism and misguided policy can impede sound public health practice."

Robert C. Gallo, MD, James P. Cullison Professor of Medicine, Director of the Institute for Translational Virology & Innovation, University of South Florida, and Co-Founder, Global Virus Network

"As a boy, I was enthralled by Paul de Kruif's *Microbe Hunters*. Reading Max Essex's memoir, *Pandemics and Politics*, is just as deeply moving and inspirational – there is no greater compliment. Essex takes us on a rousing journey across pathogens, geography, and time. His life's work is a model not only for young scientists, but for policymakers and science readers worldwide. We all owe him a profound debt of gratitude – not just for this magnificent book, but for making our world a safer, fairer place."

Lawrence Gostin, Distinguished University Professor and Founding O'Neill Chair in Global Health Law, Georgetown University, and Director, WHO Collaborating Center on Global Health Law

"*Politics and Pandemics* boosts world knowledge about the causes and cures of infectious diseases in an engaging journey. From the labs of Harvard to the landscape of Africa, the reader encounters celebrated scientists, visionary political leaders, dedicated activists, Nobel laureates, and famous celebrities. A thoroughly enjoyable and informative book."

Kitty Pilgrim, Former CNN Anchor and Author of *Summer of Fire*

"Max Essex's story is a unique combination of scientific excellence, total commitment to improving the life of those most in need, integrity in all its dimensions, and perseverance throughout political challenges and bureaucratic absurdities. This book gives a rare and real-world insight into all these dimensions. A must-read for the young and old."

Peter Piot, Author of *No Time to Lose* and Professor of Global Health, London School of Hygiene & Tropical Medicine

PANDEMICS AND POLITICS

A Scientist's Memoir

Max Essex

UNIVERSITY OF
TORONTO PRESS

Aevo UTP
An imprint of University of Toronto Press
Toronto Buffalo London
utppublishing.com
Printed and bound by CPI Group (UK) Ltd, Croydon, CR0 4YY

ISBN 978-1-0498-0473-6 (cloth)
ISBN 978-1-0498-0475-0 (EPUB)
ISBN 978-1-0498-0474-3 (PDF)

Library and Archives Canada Cataloguing in Publication
Title: Pandemics and politics : a scientist's memoir / Max Essex.
Names: Essex, Myron, author
Description: Includes bibliographical references and index.
Identifiers: Canadiana (print) 20260251208 | Canadiana (ebook) 20260251453 | ISBN 9781049804736 (cloth) | ISBN 9781049804750 (EPUB) | ISBN 9781049804743 (PDF)
Subjects: LCSH: Essex, Myron. | LCSH: Microbiologists—United States—Biography. | LCSH: Viruses. | LCGFT: Autobiographies.
Classification: LCC QR31.E87 A3 2026 | DDC 579.092—dc23

Cover design: Design Pickle

The manufacturer's authorized representative in the European Union for product safety is Mare Nostrum Group B.V., Doelen 72, 4831 GR Breda, The Netherlands. Email: gpsr@mare-nostrum.co.uk.

We wish to acknowledge the land on which the University of Toronto Press operates. This land is the traditional territory of the Wendat, the Anishnaabeg, the Haudenosaunee, the Métis, and the Mississaugas of the Credit First Nation.

University of Toronto Press acknowledges the financial support of the Government of Canada, the Canada Council for the Arts, and the Ontario Arts Council, an agency of the Government of Ontario, for its publishing activities.

Canada Council for the Arts   Conseil des Arts du Canada

ONTARIO ARTS COUNCIL
CONSEIL DES ARTS DE L'ONTARIO
an Ontario government agency
un organisme du gouvernement de l'Ontario

Funded by the Government of Canada   Financé par le gouvernement du Canada   Canada

For Elizabeth

Contents

Illustrations

Preface

It is New Year's Day, 2023, near Christiansted, St. Croix. I awake at 4 am with paroxysmal coughing and difficult breathing. The night before, New Year's Eve, I felt fine. I had only one beer to celebrate, so it isn't a hangover. My wife and I are at a lovely seacoast villa about 10 houses away from President Biden, who, by chance, is on the same island for the holiday. Elizabeth, my wife, seems concerned. She runs a COVID test. It rapidly comes up as a strong positive. At 83 and with previous heart issues and asthma, I wonder if my time is up. I take no solace in the knowledge that the COVID Omicron virus, presumably the one I'm infected with, was initially discovered by a former student, Sikhulile Moyo, in a lab I established in Botswana.

About 8 months earlier, I was in Greece. A physician colleague and friend, Shahin Lockman, had suggested I take a COVID drug with me in case I needed it and couldn't get it there. This drug was particularly important for me. I wasn't supposed to take the standard drug, Paxlovid, because it has a deleterious drug–drug interaction with another drug I was taking to prevent clotting. The COVID drug I needed, molnupiravir, was particularly difficult to find outside the United States. I didn't need a COVID drug while in Greece, but I sure did now, and fortunately I still had it with me. The molnupiravir seemed to work wonders, and within a day, all serious signs and symptoms were behind me.

This episode made me reflect on my career in virus research and my concerns about the worldwide epidemics of HIV/AIDS and

COVID. Our ability to rapidly make good drugs and vaccines has improved immensely. Fear, prejudice, global inequities, and denialism still dominate as political polarization interferes with implementation of constructive public health policy that could better protect the population. Indeed, it seems to me to have gotten worse. I think of my friends Tony Fauci at the National Institutes of Health (NIH) and Deborah Birx at the White House and all they had to contend with as they tried to do the right thing. I recall some of the governmental and societal leaders I knew during the AIDS epidemic who showed major leadership, such as President Mandela of South Africa, Presidents Mogae and Masire of Botswana, President Diouf of Senegal, President Geingob of Namibia, Princess Diana of the United Kingdom, and Princess Chulabhorn of Thailand. Such political leadership has been lacking during the time of COVID.

This book is a memoir that covers about 50 years of my career as a professor of virology at Harvard University. My laboratory research began with two cancer viruses of cats. It soon moved on to two cancer viruses of people, the hepatitis B virus and the human T cell leukemia virus. We learned that the feline leukemia virus and the human leukemia virus also caused immune suppression. This then led me, and independently Bob Gallo, to propose that a related virus might be the cause of the new epidemic of AIDS. Soon HIV/AIDS would change the world as expanding waves of disease and death confronted political leaders who were unwilling to lead.

About 40 years later, a new virus would emerge to cause another pandemic of disease and destruction. Our political systems would again become confused and overwhelmed. COVID research yielded rapid results and soon a vaccine, but too little effective public health policy. More recently, misinformation about vaccines has become commonplace, and institutions such as the US Centers for Disease Control and Prevention (CDC) have been decimated.

There will be another pandemic, probably soon. It could be even worse than the last two. Hopefully, we will experience an awakening about the importance of research and public health policy before it is too late.

Acknowledgments

Some time ago, my wife Elizabeth urged me to write something for our grandchildren about my experience during the pandemic of HIV/AIDS. She wasn't suggesting a book, just an essay about how it affected our lives. I agreed but kept postponing the assignment. When I finally began writing, it was hard to stop. Telling my story became a release for years of pent-up thoughts and emotions about the challenges posed and the frustration experienced. This book is the result.

Over almost 50 years with Harvard University, I taught numerous students – undergraduates, doctoral students, and postdoctoral research fellows – who, in truth, taught me far more than they likely realized. Some, like Phyllis Kanki, Tun-Hou Lee, Shahin Lockman, Yichen Lu, Ric Marlink, Vlad Novitsky, and Roger Shapiro, remained at Harvard as colleagues, to my good fortune. I am deeply grateful for their friendship and support. I also thank Mary Fran McLane, who managed my research lab, and Lendsey Melton, who managed everything else. Lendsey also provided invaluable assistance with the preparation of this manuscript.

From my own postdoctoral experience in Stockholm, I learned the immense value of international collaboration. I remain especially thankful for my research colleague friends in Senegal (Souleymane Mboup and Tidiane Siby), Thailand (Pornchai Matangkasombut), Botswana (Simani Gaseitsiwe, Ria Madison, Joe Makhema, Mompati Mmalane, Sikhulile Moyo, and Ibou Thior), and Tanzania (Saidi Kapiga).

The AIDS pandemic was horrific – particularly for patients, their families, and their communities. In the early years, before the cause was identified, fear was widespread and deeply personal. Virologists like me felt enormous pressure to find the cause and, ultimately, effective measures for treatment and prevention. Finding the cause of AIDS took about 3 years, but it took more than a decade before we had effective treatment and two or three decades before solutions were available for much of the world, especially Africa. The long hours, frequent travel, and workplace stress impacted us but also our families, in my case, my wife Elizabeth and my daughters Holly and Carrie. It is because of this support and the lifetime of encouragement and love that this suggestion from my wife allowed me to remember and document my life's work.

Esmond Harmsworth was a friend who was also my agent for this book. I, and many others, were devastated when he died unexpectedly in 2025, leaving a young family. I am grateful for my memories of him and all he did for me. I also thank Todd Shuster, my new agent at Aevitas, for coming to the rescue and Lohit Jagwani for supporting me at the University of Toronto Press. During the preparation of this manuscript, some friends and family also provided important advice. They included Jonathan Ball, Paul Bookbinder, Clair Chenard, Kenton Clymer, Sue Cotter, Carrie Essex, Elizabeth Essex, Bob Gallo, Bill Hardy, Bill Haseltine, Steve O'Brien, Dick Segall, Holly Steiger, Tonya Villafana, and Carolyn Wester.

Finally, I want to acknowledge the many researchers, clinicians, public health workers, and other professionals who devote their lives – sometimes at great personal cost – to protecting humanity from infectious diseases. Their work is demanding, sometimes dangerous, and too often unappreciated. The progress described in this book also depended on sustained international collaboration and the commitment of nations to support global health efforts. These partnerships remain essential. The continued strength of public health will depend on the next generation of scientists and caregivers choosing this vital path, even as they confront the consequences of weakened global cooperation, reduced financial support for research, and the growing challenges posed by anti-science misinformation.

chapter one

Mexico and the Venezuelan Encephalitis Virus

June 1964 in Catemaco, Mexico, was a special time and place. It was my introduction to research in the epidemiology of infectious diseases. It was also when I met my future wife, Elizabeth Jordan. We were both veterinary students, though in different schools – she at Cornell and I at Michigan State University. A mutual friend from Rhode Island, where I had grown up, also knew her as a Cornell classmate. Perhaps knowing that we were both interested in travel adventures, he independently suggested to us both that we apply for summer research fellowships to participate in a large project in Mexico to study the migration of Venezuelan equine encephalitis (VEE) virus.

The program was sponsored by the Pan American Health Organization, a regional affiliate of the United Nations World Health Organization. It was directed by Dr. Bill Scherer, an internationally known expert on mosquito-borne togaviruses based at Cornell University Medical College in New York City. The goal was to determine the prevalence of VEE in southern Mexico and to ascertain whether the virus was spreading north. Togaviruses were known to infect a wide range of hosts. Some were called equine encephalitis viruses because of their effects on horses, but they could also be deadly for people. The eastern equine encephalitis (EEE) virus was feared in some parts of the United States because it caused sporadic but frequently fatal human cases.

I spent my first day on the project in a sub-basement of the Cornell Medical College organizing and packing supplies and equipment for the trip. The next day, I was to fly on Aeronaves de México to Mexico City. It would be my first time outside the United States as well as my first flight. The departure was delayed twice, once for almost 10 hours after an aborted start during acceleration on the runway. Most of my fellow travelers were then reluctant to go and postponed their flight. Excited to begin my adventure, I stayed aboard and landed in Mexico City the next day. There I met Dr. Robert Dickerman, a junior faculty member and ornithologist from Cornell who had been a key leader on a similar research expedition the year before.

After packing the jeep, we drove southeast to Veracruz. The auto trip seemed even more exciting than the flight as we drove over Mount Orizaba, the third-highest mountain in North America at 18,500 feet. Starting in snow, cold, and wind, we followed a narrow switchback road with numerous crosses at each hairpin turn, ending in hot desert terrain. When crosses were above the tree line, I wondered how far the errant vehicle might have fallen while rolling down the mountain. We spent the night in a modest roadhouse after a dinner of shrimp, rice, and Dos Equis beer.

The next day, we drove through San Andrés Tuxtla to Catemaco and the Playa Azul. The hotel was modest but more than adequate to accommodate us as a base camp for the next 3 months. It had a swimming pool that often appeared to be a luxurious soup of green algae. Once a week, it was drained and scrubbed by workers, then refilled with lake water. It seemed that local labor was less expensive than a modest dose of chlorine.

For the research program, each student fellow was assigned to a subproject. Mine was birds. I was to catch both resident and migrating species of wild birds that might be spreading the virus. After driving to a forested area below the adjacent volcanic mountain range, we would look for open channels in the jungle canopy. I then used a machete to cut trails in the ground vegetation and installed invisible mist nets to capture the birds as they flew. The project director suggested that we purchase kangaroo skin boots before leaving for Mexico to work in the jungle. He said kangaroo leather was the only thing that would protect against bites from poisonous snakes that we'd encounter. I wore the boots the first day, then reverted to sneakers, as the boots seemed to impede my mobility. I saw quite a few snakes, but most were in the tall bushes or trees, well above the knee-length boots.

Each morning, I'd collect birds from the net, determine their species, collect a blood sample, and often let them go. A subset of birds were sacrificed, and a homogenate of selected internal organs was filtered and injected into the brains of neonatal mice maintained in our mobile field lab. If the mice got sick or died a few days later, it was likely to be VEE. The mice were checked for viral antigens, and the bird blood was checked for antibodies. We captured thousands of birds representing more than 200 species. About 1% were positive for VEE.[1]

Elizabeth's project was to collect and identify different species of mosquitoes. Some were harvested from conventional light traps. Others were collected by local men who were instructed to stand in the sugarcane fields with no shirt and to suction off biting mosquitoes with a small rubber hose attached to a glass tube. The young men were paid according to the number of mosquitoes they collected. They were obviously at increased risk for infection with VEE.

Later in life, I was often designing research projects that involved human trials and human sample collection while studying hepatitis B virus or human immunodeficiency virus (HIV). Our first concern then was always the ethics of doing research with human subjects and whether Harvard's Human Subjects Committee would approve our design. Had such committees been in effect in 1964, they probably would not have approved the policy of paying young men to expose themselves to disease-carrying mosquitoes by standing half-naked in swamps and fields.

The collected mosquitoes were then categorized by species, using a dissecting microscope. High-value subsets, such as those collected from human bites and known to be able to carry VEE, were also then crushed, filtered, and injected into mouse brains.[2]

Other researchers in the project were responsible for collecting blood samples from farm animals or any wild mammals that could be caught. Laboratory hamsters were also used as sentinels. They were placed in cages of wire that would allow mosquitoes in, and the cages were placed on poles in swamps where the mosquitoes bred. The hamsters were checked at frequent intervals for illness or death. If either occurred, the hamsters would be brought back to the field lab to do further analysis for VEE. The practice of using sentinel hamsters for this purpose was first developed by this group. It is probably the most sensitive way to detect endemic VEE.[3] Collection of blood samples from local people was also done. For both farm animals and people, febrile or sick individuals were given high priority. We grew to think of VEE as a ubiquitous virus that might infect almost any warm-blooded creature.

One week, three of us went on an expedition to a small village of indigenous Nahua Aztec people deep in the jungle of southeastern Mexico. We first drove to the ocean, then took a small boat up the coast as flying fish jumped around us. About 2 hours up a large river, we met a local guide who provided us with horses for a 4-hour ride through the jungle. We carried machetes and a few other tools, medical supplies, and ice packs. My horse had only a wooden saddle, which was very uncomfortable, but the slow trek was exhilarating. The path was narrow and overgrown with tangled masses of vines. Agitated herons and egrets flew above us, howler monkeys screeched, and ground mammals scampered away as we traveled through the forest. We eventually arrived in a clearing surrounded by banana trees. The settlement had several large huts with bamboo walls, dirt floors, and thatched roofs.

The village had about 40 people of all ages. Upon arrival, our leader, Dr. Scherer, met with the senior decision-maker of the village, while the rest of us, on both sides, waited in anticipation. It soon became clear that the villagers would welcome us and willingly participate in the study. The first activity was to collect blood samples from the people. With the chief going first, it seemed that all the others lined up to participate without hesitation. Apparently, their leader knew enough Spanish to communicate with Dr. Scherer, whereas most of the residents spoke only their tribal language.

After a long day, we were then treated to a dinner of corn, chicken, tortillas, and barbecued agouti, a large rodent that was common in the area. We all ate together in one of the large huts. Since we had no common language for verbal communication, we smiled but said nothing. We then moved to another hut for sleeping. It had many cots of laced bamboo, most of them wide enough for two or three people. During the night, I felt something large pushing on my cot from below. I soon discovered it was a resident pig, scratching his back. Along with other farm animals and chickens, the pigs had free access to the common sleeping hut.

The next morning, after a breakfast of tea, bananas, and some unknown meat, we took blood samples from the village animals, including chickens, pigs, goats, and the horses that brought us there. We stored the blood samples on ice, gave our thanks with several gifts, and rode the horses back to our small boat at the river bank. Upon returning to base camp, I was sore and exhausted but thrilled with the experience.

Several years after we completed our fellowships, scientific papers were published on many aspects of the project. Most of the fellows, like me, had an opportunity to co-author one of our first publications.[1–3]

VEE outbreaks were later documented in Texas and Florida, verifying our concerns about northward migration. Some species of transmitter mosquitoes not previously seen in the United States became established in the Everglades, perhaps as another aspect of global warming. Although VEE is not as lethal in adults as the EEE that was already here, VEE could still kill a third or more of young children who became infected.

VEE also provides a vivid illustration of some of the principles of "spillover," where viruses that remain endemic in animal species may occasionally move to people if contact between the different species occurs. With COVID or SARS, such spillover may have occurred in the wet markets, where workers were butchering civets or racoon dogs, or perhaps, in the case of COVID, when lab workers were growing viruses harvested from wild bats that are highly infected in nature. To identify SARS-related viruses that might grow more effectively in cultured cells, a lab worker might become accidentally infected and then start a new epidemic in people. For SARS, COVID, and other related viruses, large colonies of infected bats in caves have probably evolved to resist death or serious disease from the infection. Periodically, the virus could spill over to palm civets, racoon dogs, or ferret-badgers when these species get attacked by a viremic bat.[4] The origin of the SARS-related viruses is discussed in greater detail in chapter 15.

For VEE, the equivalent of the endemic populations of infected bats are mice or wild birds. While respiratory aerosol transmission may be necessary for SARS or COVID, mosquitoes regularly move VEE virus within feral mouse or bird populations. Occasionally, when the mosquitoes bite horses or people, spillover occurs. If a horse becomes highly viremic, mosquitoes moving from horses to people may become particularly dangerous. Unlike COVID, however, the risk of VEE moving directly from one person to another would be negligible because of the need for a mosquito vector.

This introduction to VEE research, combined with my ensuing education in veterinary or comparative medicine, helped provide me both the background and initiative to study future epidemics like HIV/AIDS. It also taught me the importance of an interdisciplinary approach when trying to understand epidemics and stimulated me to continue to study viruses.

chapter two

Michigan and California

We got married in June 1966. Elizabeth graduated with her doctorate of veterinary medicine (DVM), passed her board exams, and finished the final arrangements for our wedding to occur during the same week. We then went on a brief honeymoon to eat lobster on the coast of Maine and drove to Michigan so I could complete my degrees.

After I graduated from the University of Rhode Island with a bachelor's degree in biology in 1962, I decided I wanted to be a medical scientist. I thought that domestic animals with infectious diseases, cancer, or genetic abnormalities provided researchers with good models to help us understand comparable diseases in people. When Michigan State offered support to do both a master of science/doctorate (MS/PhD) and a DVM at the same time, I thought that would be the best track. I was known among my vet school classmates as the only one they knew who went to vet school with no intention of becoming a veterinarian. Even if I had considered veterinary practice, I would soon have ruled it out when I found I was allergic to cats and horses. But that shouldn't matter if I were just doing laboratory research. For my MS/PhD program, I selected microbiology. Scientific news reports about cancer-causing viruses in mice and chickens were becoming more common, and there was speculation about cancers that could be prevented or reversed by immune responses.

My thesis topic was crib death, a rare and mysterious condition where infants are found dead with no logical explanation.

The hypotheses about cause ranged from a respiratory infection to a psychotic reaction by the mother. My hypothesis was that the infant might develop an allergic reaction to cow's milk, which would produce an anaphylactic shock that could be lethal.[5]

My thesis advisor maintained a research facility that housed gnotobiotic animals, especially mice. It was initially established by delivering baby mice, using Caesarean section in a sterile incubator, and then maintaining them in a large, plastic bubble-like enclosure. They were then regularly checked to be sure they were free of all known microbes on skin and oral mucosa, and in the gut. All food and water for the animals had to be sterilized and carefully brought into the bubble through a controlled sterile channel. After the mice matured, they gave birth by natural means for the next generation and all future generations, never leaving the sterile environment and checked often for contaminants. For experiments, single species of bacteria or viruses or immunogens could be introduced alone or together to examine their effects in the absence of other contaminating species. Similarly, we could clearly examine immune responses to microbial antigens or potential allergens to determine how a purified body might respond. Even by the 1960s, it was known that some bacterial proteins could act as adjuvants, enhancing immune responses to other things.

The mice in my experiments developed immune responses to milk proteins, but in the end, that didn't move us much closer to understanding crib death. More than 50 years later, we still don't understand much about the cause of crib death, though it has been determined that placing infants on their back, rather than their stomach, reduces the risk, presumably by keeping airways open.

While in Michigan, I was involved in two serious accidents. In neither was I a driver nor even in an auto. The first happened just a couple of months after I arrived in 1962. While walking to class across East Grand River Avenue, I was struck from behind by a car. It resulted in fractures in three pelvic bones. I was hospitalized for about 4 months, the first 2 months locked in full-body compression with a Stryker frame that rotated every 2–3 hours. It was 7 or 8 months before I could walk without crutches.

The second accident was even worse. It happened a few months after Elizabeth and I arrived back at Michigan State after getting married. We moved into a small ground-floor apartment in Lansing. We were referred to the apartment by a vet school classmate and friend from Rhode Island, Bruce Remor, who lived in the apartment above us. He often traveled to class, about 6 miles away, on a motor scooter. One day, he invited me to ride with him, and I accepted, riding behind him on the back of the seat. I had a flash of a head-on collision and later awoke in the Lansing Hospital. Bruce was killed instantly. According to a witness, I glanced off him and over the car, landing on the sidewalk. For his family, it was horrendous. His wife, Barbara, was a nurse at the hospital where the ambulance brought him in. His parents were en route from Rhode Island to Michigan to visit their newborn grandchild and learned upon arrival that their son was dead.

In 1966, my thesis advisor accepted a job at Ohio State University, leaving me in the position of needing to find a new advisor and a new project for my PhD thesis if I stayed at Michigan State. I could continue with him if we moved to Ohio State. Alternatively, by the time I finished vet school in 9 months, I'd be eligible for a larger postdoctoral-level stipend if I did the PhD at another institution. So we decided to leave Michigan and follow the flower children to California. My MS thesis was typed by Elizabeth on a manual typewriter, and we moved to the University of California at Davis (UCD), where I was enrolled in a PhD program and Elizabeth would be an intern in the small animal clinic at the veterinary school.

The late 1960s and the early 1970s saw significant increases in funding for medical research. Perhaps the greatest increase was for cancer research, following diagnoses of cancer in a few elderly senators on key committees. Mary Lasker, whom I'd eventually get to know some 20 years later, was often credited for her lobbying of Congress to fund a massive expansion of the National Institutes of Health (NIH), especially the National Cancer Institute (NCI). This led to the Special Virus Cancer Program and the National Cancer Act. Often compared to President John F. Kennedy's space mission that led a successful moon landing in 1969, the rapid funding and mobilization of scientific expertise was sometimes called President

Richard Nixon's "War on Cancer." Among the many new projects was a program at UCD to look for new cancer viruses in different species of domestic animals.

RNA tumor viruses had already been found in chickens and, in the late 1950s and 1960s, in several strains of laboratory mice.[6] Some mouse strains with the most evident cancer viruses had actually been bred for the phenotype of death from leukemia or breast cancer. Nonetheless, this caused some scientists, medical journalists, and politicians to speculate that human tumor viruses would still be found. Many labs examined human cancer cells for "virus-like particles" using such techniques as ultra-high magnification electron microscopy and searches for cross-reactive antibodies that would react with the mouse viruses. It would be more than a decade before any RNA-type tumor viruses would be found in humans. But there were several false alarms along the way, where the newly discovered human viruses turned out to be laboratory contaminants, usually mouse viruses.

The study of mouse and chicken viruses did, however, yield a breakthrough in molecular biology with the discovery in 1970 of reverse transcriptase by Howard Temin[7] and David Baltimore,[8] whom I would later know as colleagues. Both received Nobel Prizes for this work in 1975. Until their discovery, it was assumed that DNA could not be made from RNA. Although their research was done to try to understand cancer, this discovery also gave rise to much of the biotechnology industry and to such things as the use of forensic DNA in solving crimes.

My PhD project at UCD was part of a larger program to find viruses in cancer cells of animals such as cats, dogs, and cattle. At the veterinary school, there was an abundance of cancer tissues from these common domestic animal species and finely tuned diagnoses of the cancers by veterinary oncologists and pathologists. Students and postdoctoral fellows, including myself, spent hours scanning suspect cancer tissues. This took more than the usual commitment to laboratory work, as the facility housing the electron microscope was infested with black widow spiders.

At least three new tumor viruses, the feline sarcoma virus,[9] the gibbon ape leukemia virus,[10] and the woolly monkey sarcoma virus,[11] were discovered in our lab in the brief time I was there, though none by me. In that era, viruses were often named after the person who first described them. So the feline sarcoma virus, discovered by fellow graduate student Stan Snyder, became known as the Snyder-Theilen virus.

The feline leukemia virus (FeLV) had been discovered a few years earlier by Dr. Bill Jarrett, a pathologist at the University of Glasgow veterinary school.[12] The discovery of FeLV was confirmed and extended by Dr. Tom Kawakami, a biophysicist at UCD, who used some new techniques to find RNA tumor viruses.[13] Because each group of viruses has unique physical properties of size, shape, and density, he used ultracentrifugation through sensitive chemical gradients to detect, concentrate, and purify the viruses. With compounds like cesium chloride or even selected concentrations of sucrose, one could add substances like blood plasma and, following ultracentrifugation, test the band where RNA tumor viruses would be expected to migrate. Other RNA tumor viruses, like the mouse tumor viruses, could be used as a positive control. The viruses could then be sorted according to their buoyant density or even their sedimentation coefficient, which was based on the speed at which the virus moved through the gradient. Kawakami extended the technology to allow the sieving of large volumes of blood plasma through gradients based on "continuous flow" techniques. I was impressed with Kawakami and chose him as my PhD thesis advisor.

For my thesis research, I studied the host range of the FeLV to see if it would grow in other cells beyond leukemic lymphocytes and whether it would grow in cells from other species, including those of canine, porcine, and human origin. I also developed a new serological test to rapidly determine if different cells were infected, along with a new test to see how much virus the different types of infected cells could produce. We found that cells other than blood lymphocytes, such as lung epithelial cells, could be easily infected, raising the possibility of oral transmission. Surprisingly, cells from species other than cats, including human cells, could also be easily infected. I also found that the FeLV would grow in other types of cells, like epithelium, raising the possibility of mucosal transmission. This raised the theoretical concern that such viruses might be transmitted to people, but that possibility was greatly reduced when samples from people of high risk were always negative for FeLV. In retrospect, after recent public health concerns about the possibility that COVID might have originated from a lab accident with an animal virus grown in human cells, my studies with FeLV grown in human cells might now seem inappropriate or unnecessarily risky. All such studies we conducted were, however, done in a negative-pressure biocontainment laboratory designed for high-risk research.

During this time period, there was a massive expansion of our knowledge in molecular biology and genetics. The first wave came with knowledge of how some viruses infected bacteria and then copied their own genes along with the replicating bacteria. The double helix structure had long been established by Watson and Crick.[14] RNA synthesis from DNA, or transcription, was also then described and, soon after, specific proteins composed of amino acids could then be translated from the messenger RNA. Two additional discoveries paved the way for a revolution in molecular biology and biotechnology. The first was the discovery of a way to rapidly sequence DNA by Dr. Wally Gilbert at Harvard.[15] The second was the development of polymerase chain reaction (PCR) by Dr. Kary Mullis.[16] This allowed the rapid amplification of DNA so it could be categorized and matched to known sequences. These techniques are what allow us to recognize viral variants and classify them as new strains with minor differences or as entirely new viruses. It seems ironic that both Mullis and Gilbert would later become skeptics or denialists about human immunodeficiency virus (HIV) being the cause of AIDS. Students like me sometimes developed reverence for such accomplished senior scientists. This was a reminder that even great scientists could be wrong.

Many tumor viruses were also being discovered. Dr. Tony Epstein, a British pathologist, discovered that Burkitt lymphoma, an aggressive form of non-Hodgkin's lymphoma, was regularly associated with a type of herpes virus. This was subsequently called the Epstein-Barr virus (EBV).[17] EBV was shown to be the cause of infectious mononucleosis and linked to other cancers like nasopharyngeal carcinoma. Other herpes viruses would also be associated with cancers like Kaposi sarcoma.[18] Among the most interesting were herpes saimiri in squirrel monkeys and herpes ateles in spider monkeys.[19] Surprisingly, these viruses were usually present in their native species, squirrel or spider monkeys, in the absence of disease. But if the viruses were injected into other species of monkeys, the viruses would induce an acute and fatal leukemia or lymphoma. This raised many questions about how these species evolved to avoid the lethal effects that the viruses clearly possessed. One likely possibility seemed to be that some species of monkeys have undergone a process of genetic selection for survival through many generations. One way the naturally resistant monkeys might express protection could be with an active immune response. By this time, immunity was also known to be mediated by immune response genes. For a protective immune response to the herpes virus–induced leukemia, it seemed there could be two potential targets: the virus itself and the cells that were made leukemic by the virus.

As time went on, I became convinced that the feline leukemia and sarcoma viruses provided an excellent model to study how immunosurveillance of a cancer might occur. Even before going to UCD, I had been impressed with the research and theories of Dr. George Klein, who was head of the Department of Tumor Biology at the Karolinska Institute in Stockholm, Sweden, and thought it would be great to learn from him. Elizabeth was also enthusiastic about the possibility of going to Stockholm for a couple of years.

Our first child, Holly Anne, was born in 1969 in Woodland, California. She was a gorgeous baby. I soon learned that I could get her to sleep most easily by holding her on my chest while I lay on our small living room floor. While I couldn't write in this position, I could effectively read scientific papers, journals, and lab results, while organizing thoughts for writing my thesis.

A new challenge I faced was to find financial support for a fellowship in Stockholm. After corresponding with Dr. Klein about my interests, I met him at a cancer conference in Houston in 1969. He encouraged me to join his group but said I would have to obtain my own fellowship for financial support if I were to begin research there on the cat viruses rather than with the mouse system for which he already had funded research grants. With his endorsement, I submitted my first research proposal to three different funding agencies. I was pleasantly surprised when they were all successful, and I chose the grant from the Leukemia Society of America because it also offered the possibility of applying for future research support following completion of the 2-year fellowship period. After a brief visit to New York and Rhode Island so our families could meet Holly, we were off to Sweden.

chapter three

Stockholm

In late summer of 1970, we flew from New York to Stockholm. After landing at Arlanda Airport, we rode about an hour south to the northern edge of the city, ending at the Wenner-Gren Center, where we would live. The Wenner-Gren Center included a horseshoe-shaped three-story building with about 50 furnished apartments. It seemed luxurious with two bedrooms and two baths, and only a 20-minute walk or short bus ride to downtown Stockholm. The Wenner-Gren was also adjacent to Haga Park, an outdoor forest of woodland walking trails, and to an inlet of the Bothnian Sea. In winter, the sea was securely frozen, and it was said you could skate all the way to Finland. I never tried. The center was built specifically to provide low-cost housing to accommodate foreign scientists and scholars at the universities and research institutes of Stockholm. It seemed perfect for us. It was about a 15-minute walk for me to go across a small section of Haga Park, then across the large hospital complex, to get to the Department of Tumor Biology at the Karolinska Institute Medical School where I'd be based. Elizabeth attended clinical conferences at the Swedish Veterinary School in Stockholm.

We soon began to recognize some of the benefits of the socialized government system. When Holly had a severe case of croup, she was hospitalized overnight at the pediatrics wing of the Karolinska with intubation and appropriate medication. The total cost was 2 kronor, about 45 cents. Each year, the government sent us and all families, whether citizens or foreign visitors, a stipend to care for young children. Each section of the city had a daycare facility where you could leave preschool-aged children at no cost.

My mentor, Dr. George Klein, was the professor in charge of the department. There were about 8 other faculty-level researchers and at least 20 others like myself at some level of research training, and probably another 30 support staff. The scientists in training were from all corners of the world – a few from the United States and more than a few from Sweden, but others were from the USSR, Argentina, England, Japan, Germany, Yugoslavia, Kenya, Italy, and Israel, just to name a few. English was the common language for the building. I began to learn Swedish but found I really didn't need it. Everyone in the research group seemed to be culturally cosmopolitan and cordial, which was refreshing. It left me with the feeling that, when I eventually had my own lab group, I'd want it to be very international.

George Klein was a renaissance man in his interests and expertise. He was recognized and respected for his accomplishments in disciplines ranging from radiation biology and biochemistry to virology and immunology, while his focus was on cancer research. He was an author of more than a thousand research publications and at least a dozen books. He spoke many languages. He was also one who avoided all customs of status associated with academic royalty. One time when I rode with him to the airport, the driver addressed him as Professor Klein. His reply was, "I don't use that title; you must call me George." His dress was very casual, perhaps even deliberately dull. His wife, Eva, also an accomplished scientist, bought all his clothes. I recall one time when she bought him a dozen identical pairs of shoes. She mentioned that they fit him very well, so she wouldn't have to buy him any more shoes in his lifetime. I knew both George and Eva were from Hungary. I later learned that, as a teenager, he escaped from a train deporting Jews from Budapest to the Auschwitz concentration camp.[20] George took pride in multitasking. He dictated scientific correspondence while examining fluorescing cancer cells under a microscope. He read scientific papers while jogging on campus, which occasionally resulted in his running into a parked car.

The lab was crowded well beyond normal capacity. All the equipment was shared. I shared an office desk with two others, one being Hans Wigzell, who would become a world-renowned immunologist in his own right and later go on to become president of both the University of Uppsala and the Karolinska Institute. Most researchers worked long hours and late into the night. I soon learned that I could get much better access to the biohazard hoods and ultracentrifuges if I arrived very early, like 5 or 6 am. Most of the others didn't arrive until 9 or 10 am after staying until midnight the day before. Arriving early was easy to do in the spring and summer, when the "midnight sun" provided so much light, but harder in the cold, dark winter. Starting early became a habit that I'd follow for the rest of my career.

The Swedes seemed to work even harder in the winter, perhaps to preserve their time off for the long days of summer. But even the dark days of December seemed fascinating to Elizabeth and me. It started with the Nobel Prize ceremonies in early December, a very elegant event with presentations by the King at the Stockholm Concert Hall and then the banquet at the City Hall, an impressive structure of Venetian Gothic style. The recipients of the Nobel Prize in Medicine and Physiology were selected by the senior faculty of the Karolinska. In 1970, George Klein was the chair of the committee, which explained why we were invited. That year was particularly suspenseful as Aleksandr Solzhenitsyn, the Russian dissident, won the prize in literature. Everyone was anxiously awaiting to see if the Soviet government would let him out to receive the award. They didn't.

Nobel week was soon followed by St. Lucia Day. Traditionally a major celebration in Sweden on December 13, the winter solstice, the "festival of lights" was to mark the beginning of the Christmas season. The eldest daughter would dress in white with a wreath of candles on her head while serving coffee and saffron bread to the rest of the family. As a toddler, Holly was too young to appreciate her ceremonial role, but we all enjoyed the festivities.

Overall, the food was a mixed bag. We loved the pepparkakor cookies, Swedish meatballs, crayfish, and green marzipan cakes. But we could have done without the pickled herring, lutefisk, and blood pudding, which was the regular Wednesday lunch at the Karolinska cafeteria. The chicken was tough and beef too expensive, but the horse meat was good, both as loin steaks and in sliced deli sandwiches.

In the 1960s, Klein was a world leader on the theory of immunosurveillance – that the immune response could be mobilized to attack and destroy cancer cells. He was probably way ahead of his time. Forty to 50 years later, immune therapy would be a tool in the regimens of clinical oncologists, at least those at major cancer centers. By 1970, it was already apparent that cancers caused by viruses might provide the best way to understand the mechanisms involved. It seemed to me that the feline leukemia and sarcoma viral systems would be an ideal way to advance our knowledge about immune mechanisms that might work against both leukemia and solid tumors. Klein's lab already had developed immune assays for both the murine leukemia virus system and for Burkitt lymphoma in people. One of the most valuable tests was a way to look at the membrane surface of cancer cells with immunofluorescence using antibodies from mouse or human cancer survivors. We sought to set up the same type of assay with cultured leukemia cells from cats that were infected with either the feline leukemia virus (FeLV) and/or the feline sarcoma virus (FeSV).

FeLV and FeSV are closely related. In fact, FeSV is a hybrid virus that contains most of the genes of FeLV along with a newly inserted cancer gene that can transform muscle cells to make them cancerous. The newly acquired transformation gene could also make the FeSV defective for self-replication, so it usually needed FeLV to replicate along with it.

We used blood serum samples from cats infected with FeSV to measure the correlation between immune antibodies and progression of the tumors. Cats that developed either no tumors or tumors that subsequently regressed had high levels of antibodies, whereas cats that had lethal progressing tumors failed to develop measurable levels of the same antibodies. Our study, published in the journal *Nature*, seemed to be a good example of immune attack because the killer antibodies were directed at the surfaces of cancer cells.[21] In a related study, we found that young kittens, whose immune mothers had antibodies to the cancer cell membrane antigens, were themselves protected against tumor development when exposed to FeSV. The antibodies in the kittens were presumably transmitted through the mothers' milk. The antibodies also seemed to protect against both solid tumor sarcomas and leukemias.[22] Hyperimmune serum taken from resistant adults could also be used to prevent tumors by passive administration to unprotected cats in much the same way that immune serum to rabies can be used to protect people exposed to a bite by a rabid animal. Subsequently, we studied cats in multiple-cat households where one or more cats had developed leukemia as a natural disease. Among the healthy cats who did not develop leukemia in the same households, most had protective antibodies. Overall, this appeared to be a good example of immunosurveillance against cancer.[23]

By midsummer of 1971, we had earned a holiday. We purchased a Volkswagen camper that we could later ship back to the United States. At the time, we would use it for low-cost travel to visit the Norwegian fjords, Great Britain, and parts of Europe en route to the International Leukemia Meeting in Venice. Eva Klein was responsible for inviting some of the speakers for the conference, and she invited me to give a presentation on immunosurveillance. It was my first speech at a scientific meeting. It went well. Dr. Gino Chieco-Bianchi, a professor at the University of Padova who was chair of the meeting, and his wife, Anna Maria, soon became lifelong friends.

After returning to Stockholm, we had to face the reality of a plan to move back to the United States and begin a career in academic teaching and research. I applied again to the Leukemia Society of America, this time for the highly competitive 5-year Scholar Award that would also provide me with a significantly higher salary. Elizabeth and I already knew that our preference would be to settle in New England, ideally in an institution with a large research base and close to our families in Rhode Island and New York. The universities in Boston were the most obvious, but we also considered the University of Vermont in Burlington and Dartmouth in New Hampshire. I had two friends who educated me about Harvard. One whom I had occasionally played tennis with at UCD had left a junior faculty position in virology at Harvard to accept a senior position in California. He believed that the position he left in Boston was still open and I could apply for that. The other who gave me some advice was George Klein. Harvard had tried to recruit him as chair of pathology. He obviously didn't go but said he was impressed by the size and quality of the research faculty on the Boston campus. So I sent letters of inquiry to the departments of microbiology at Harvard, the University of Vermont, and Dartmouth along with my curriculum vitae. The departments of microbiology at Harvard's School of Public Health and the Dartmouth Medical School got back soon with indications of interest. At about that time, I also won the Leukemia Society of America's coveted Scholar Award, which helped me immensely.

As I started negotiating from Sweden with Harvard and Dartmouth, I made an incredible mistake. My letters with requests for lab space, equipment, technical support, salary, and all the rest were somehow put into the wrong envelopes. So the letter to the Dartmouth chair was accidentally sent to Harvard and vice versa. I was shocked when I got my letter to Dartmouth sent back by the Harvard chair's secretary with a message stating, "You must have sent this by mistake." Indeed I had, and I wrote to both with apologies. I wondered if they thought I just had outsized chutzpah while trying to cover it as the stupid mistake it really was. But as soon as they realized I had other serious offers, which I had not mentioned before, my value seemed to go up even more. I took a short trip from Stockholm to Boston to look at lab space and meet potential colleagues, along with a dinner with my sister at the Hilltop Steak House. I then quickly negotiated an agreement. In early 1972, we moved to Boston as I became an assistant professor at Harvard.

chapter four

Harvard and the Multiple-Cat Households

The Harvard medical campus on Longwood Avenue in Boston is a massive enterprise. Along with the Medical School, the School of Public Health, and the Dental School are major research and teaching hospitals, such as Brigham and Women's Hospital, Beth Israel Deaconess Hospital, the Dana-Farber Cancer Institute, and Boston Children's Hospital. More than 10,000 doctoral-level professionals are appointed at the Medical School alone. A few miles across town is the Massachusetts General Hospital, and just across the Charles River, Harvard College and Massachusetts Institute of Technology (MIT). Harvard and MIT have many joint programs, including biomedical research organizations like the Broad and Ragon Institutes. The Tufts and Boston University medical schools and hospitals are also within a 5-mile radius. No place else in the world can claim such a large concentration of medical researchers within a few miles. Even if one is not impressed with quantity, the quality of the researchers at these institutions, based on awards and funding, is high. It is easy to see why a newly appointed assistant professor from outside the system, like me, might be in awe of the situation.

Upon arrival, we also had to address some very important family matters. Elizabeth was pregnant with our second child, also a girl we'd soon name Carrie Lisa. Elizabeth also wanted to get back to her work in veterinary practice as soon as possible. She found a good position at the Norwood Animal Hospital, about 20 miles from the Harvard medical campus. Her responsibilities included emergency care, so she had to work some nights and weekends, and be available to respond within 15–20 minutes. So we found a place to live in Norwood, which was close to a Boston train stop. Whether I drove or took the train, I followed my earlier pattern of going to work at 5 am. Soon after our arrival, Carrie Lisa was born at the Brigham and Women's Hospital, which was right across Longwood Avenue and my office. She was also a beautiful baby. Elizabeth and I had a busy household with two working parents, a 3-year-old, and a new infant.

The Department of Microbiology, which I joined, was in the School of Public Health. The department faculty also worked closely with the Department of Tropical Public Health through the Division of Infectious Diseases. The most senior virologist, Tom Weller, who had won a Nobel Prize for his work with poliovirus in 1954, was also head of the division. The chair of my department was Roger Nichols, whose research was on trachoma in the Middle East, especially Saudi Arabia. Just after I arrived, the School of Public Health appointed a new dean, Dr. Howard Hiatt. I mentioned this to George Klein, my mentor in Sweden, with whom I kept in close contact. George's comment was, "Oh, that's terrible, what will happen to his research?" George felt that cancer research was more important than academic administration, though it would soon become clear that Hiatt was needed to move the school ahead in the right direction.[24]

Although my own research on immunosurveillance of FeLV- and FeSV-induced tumors in cats seemed to be accepted and respected, the Special Virus Cancer Program seemed to be losing some of its vigor. More was being learned about the mouse and chicken viruses and how they transformed cells, but discoveries of new viruses in naturally occurring cancers of other species, especially people, had become stagnant. At the same time, it was clear that genetics played an important role in some human cancers.

This induced many of the "virus cancer" researchers to focus primarily on molecular mechanisms and how the mouse and chicken viruses transformed cells through oncogenes that the viruses had acquired. Enthusiasm developed for the concept that retroviruses caused cancer by genetic inheritance rather than by transmission of the infectious forms of the virus from one individual to another.[25] As more people looked for endogenous inherited retroviruses or retroviral-related DNA sequences in normal mouse or human cells, the more they found. Some activated endogenous retroviruses actually grew in cell cultures, but usually only in cells from animal species different from the species in which they were found as inherited DNA. Such viral sequences found in normal mouse DNA, for example, might grow in human or dog cells but not in mouse cells, which led to their categorization as "xenotrophs." However, it was soon discovered that such endogenous xenotropic viruses had no particular association with cancer development. It had been clearly established that all retroviruses, including FeLV, had to integrate into cellular DNA to replicate themselves, but those that caused cancer didn't stay as endogenous viruses and get passed through generations via the germ line. The latter appeared to occur for only those viruses that evolved to become non-virulent. Evolutionary selection worked against viruses that could remain in the germ line if they caused disease before the reproductive stage had ended.

Also working to diminish enthusiasm for the "virus cancer" direction was the apparent failure to find new human cancer viruses. A few were found after conducting experiments where human leukemia cells were co-cultured with mouse cells, but those putative human retroviruses, sometimes called "human rumor viruses" by the cynics, were ultimately shown to be laboratory contaminants. One NIH scientist, Dr. Bob Gallo, was especially enthusiastic about our findings with cat leukemia viruses and still believed that such viruses would eventually be found in some human leukemias. He was right. As the role of leukemic retroviruses grew more confusing for naturally occurring cancer in mice and chickens, we decided we must learn more detail about how leukemia viruses were spread among cats. Were they truly contagious viruses transmitted as infectious agents? To address this, we decided to do more studies with the population of pet housecats that had naturally occurring leukemia.

Soon after moving to Harvard, I recognized that the largest referral veterinary clinic in the state, the Angell Memorial Animal

Hospital, was a few buildings away on Longwood Avenue. Assuming they'd have quite a few cases of cat leukemia, I attended some pathology conferences there and introduced myself to Dr. Susan Cotter, a clinical veterinarian who was interested in the disease. She gave us several tips about "multiple-cat households" that also had multiple cases of cat leukemia. At the same time, I decided to reach out for collaboration with two other research groups who focused on cat leukemia. One was the lab of Dr. William Jarrett at the University of Glasgow, the same guy who had discovered the virus in 1964. The second was Dr. William Hardy, a veterinarian who had a research group at the Memorial Sloan Kettering Cancer Center in New York City. We all seemed to have common research interests, and we soon found that the benefits of collaboration were more than enough to offset the disadvantages of geographical separation.

My first introduction to a multiple-cat leukemia household was in Boston, a 600-square-foot, three-room apartment whose owner had 35 cats during the period of 1970–1973. The owner was a client of Dr. Cotter, who took me on a field trip to visit the population, which also included one person, the cat owner, and three dogs. Almost all of the cats were taken in as unrelated strays and were never allowed out after entering the house. After a quick look into the apartment, and an even quicker smell, I decided I'd have to remain outside to survive my own cat allergy. I waited patiently while Sue collected blood samples from the cats. Eleven of the cats died of leukemia during the 3-year period, most testing positive for FeLV.[26] Another four died of a type of peritonitis that was caused by a coronavirus. The cats that developed leukemia were unrelated, and relatives of the leukemic cats were no more likely to get leukemia. This was strong support for horizontal or contagious transmission of the virus. We also found that cats who developed leukemia had low levels of antibodies to the leukemic cell surface proteins, but healthy exposed cats in the same environments often had much higher levels of antibodies. This strongly supported our earlier evidence for immunosurveillance in experimental cats.

Evidence that a horizontally transmitted contagious virus could cause leukemia or any other type of cancer under natural conditions was hard for many to accept. The general understanding of infectious diseases was that the causative virus or bacterium would be transmitted by body fluids, which would be acquired by inhalation or ingestion and cause diseases like flu or gastroenteritis within a few days after exposure. Under such a scenario, the causative agent should be found quite readily by contact tracing or "shoe leather" epidemiology to determine how each case in a disease outbreak may have had recent contact with other cases that had a similar diagnosis. With smallpox, for example, worldwide eradication was achieved by simply identifying obvious cases, keeping them in quarantine or isolation for a brief period, and vaccinating all who might come in contact with them.

Cancers, on the other hand, took many months or years to develop. So if they were caused by viruses, the virus would remain in the body for many months or years before the disease would be clinically diagnosed. Some viruses, like retroviruses or herpes viruses, were able to do this. They could sometimes hide their DNA in cells without activation for replication as whole virus particles and sometimes not even make their antibody-inducing proteins. Cancer epidemiologists routinely considered that whatever first changed a normal cell into a cancer cell, whether a spontaneous mutation or an exogenous carcinogen, it probably happened long before the cancer was diagnosed. Even if disease clusters occurred, it would be hard to link the cause back to when the damage started as one or a few cancer cells years earlier.

We thought we still had much to learn about transmission and disease development in the multiple-cat households. As word got out among veterinarians about our results, our opportunities also increased. I was contacted by Dr. Richard Jakowski, a pathologist at the University of Connecticut, saying he could get access to a house in central Connecticut that had multiple cases of cat leukemia. We got our team together, which included Sue Cotter and me from Boston, along with a technician from Angell Memorial who was an expert at holding cats to collect blood samples. Bill Hardy, from New York City, and Dr. Jakowski met us at the site. Dr. Jakowski briefed us. He said he already had 10 pathologically confirmed cases of lymphocytic leukemia or lymphoma from the house over the previous 18 months. It was a nine-room house that had about 150 cats during that same period. As we got to the house, the owner pointed out two full refrigerator-sized freezers in the garage. One was filled with cat food. The other was filled with dead cats, which we moved to cardboard cat carriers for Jakowski to take back to the University of Connecticut pathology lab to do autopsies. Ironically, the only cat carriers he had for the dead animals had a printed message on the side that read "I'm feeling better now, thank you." About half of the cats were Abyssinian, and almost half were Burmese, originally from the Thai–Burma border. About 10 were domestic short hair, taken in as strays. All except one cat were confined inside. Seeing just the one domestic short hair on the front steps, neighbors and passers-by probably had no idea about the 150 others inside.

Again my allergy kept me outside the house while Sue Cotter got blood samples from 125 of the cats held on the kitchen table. Over 90% of the cats had either active infection with FeLV or former infection based on antibodies.[27] Most of the dead cats that Jakowski took back to autopsy had lymphocytic leukemia or lymphoma. There were no significant differences for percentage infected or antibody level according to breed. Even as it was clear that the virus caused the leukemia, it was hard to make a case for genetic differences based on breed. The transmission of FeLV in this and other multiple-cat households we studied was almost certainly enhanced by the crowding. Livestock veterinarians get concerned about rampant infectious diseases when animals such as pigs or cattle are concentrated in pens or feed lots. Crowded cat households presented a similar situation.

By the time we were conducting studies of multiple-cat households, we could employ a new lab test for the virus that Bill Hardy had developed. His test resulted in a high-impact publication in the journal *Nature*, convincing even the skeptics that a virus causing leukemia could be spread in a contagious manner, if only in cats.[28]

As our research opportunities expanded, I realized that I'd need more financial support to cover the laboratory expenses. Most new faculty members in my situation submitted a grant proposal to the National Institutes of Health to help pay for the research. I submitted my proposal to cover various aspects of FeLV and FeSV tumor development and potential immune control. The proposal was rejected. This was my first major disappointment with my research. Feeling frustrated and dejected, I called a friend, Dr. Satvir Tevethia, a virologist who had completed his PhD about five years before me and seemed settled as a faculty member at the Baylor School of Medicine. I knew he had some experience both submitting and reviewing NIH grant proposals. As soon as I described my situation, he tried to calm me down, saying rejection was common when new, younger faculty members made their first submission. Pending further comment, he asked that I send him the proposal and the written comments provided by the anonymous reviewers to support their decision. I sent him the review. A few days later he called. His first comment was, "This is great." I replied, "Are you crazy? They turned me down." He responded, "But the way they turned you down is great. They said your hypothesis is original, and the research you propose is important, but you propose doing too much for a first proposal. It is too ambitious." He went on to say, "This is what you should do. Thank them for their constructive review and reduce your specific aims or goals in half. Resubmit that to the same section at the NIH right away. Then take the other half of the original proposal and submit it to the American Cancer Society." I followed his very wise advice and was soon ecstatic to find that both proposals were approved and funded for a total of almost twice as much money as I had asked for with the first NIH proposal a few months before. It was a dramatic lesson on the importance of grantsmanship.

The new grant money could be used to purchase research equipment and hire technicians and students. I needed new biohazard negative-pressure hoods to protect lab workers, including myself, who were handling concentrated virus; a newer ultracentrifuge so I could concentrate the virus more effectively; and a couple of chest freezers so I could effectively store our growing stocks of cat blood samples and purified viruses. I had one freezer that was left in the lab following the departure of the former virologist occupant. But the freezer had a large box of frozen material in plastic bags. On closer examination, this material looked like human feet. The box had a label inside saying that the enclosed feet were collected for Dr. Maurice Hilleman at the Merck Institute for Research. Hilleman, whom I knew, was an eminent scientist responsible for the development of most human vaccines, like measles, mumps, and rubella. I called Maurice. He said they were indeed human feet, and he'd like to get them. He explained that the feet were dug up in northern Alaska where the graves indicated the death was that of a young person who died during the flu epidemic of 1918. It was only feet because of the manner of burial. Below 30 inches was a thick layer of permafrost that was difficult to penetrate, especially with the lack of mechanized equipment at that time. The dead bodies would be bent at the knees and a large enough hole dug in the ice to anchor the feet. The rest of the body would be covered with unfrozen dirt. After many decades, the permanently frozen feet should be well-preserved, even though the rest of the body had decayed and washed away due to annual thawing. He felt that some viable flu viruses from the 1918 epidemic might still be found in the feet. Even if they weren't viable, the viral genomes might still be salvaged. Modern techniques for gene amplification and sequencing would probably allow a comparison of the 60-year-old flu virus to contemporary strains circulating in the current epidemics. I sent Maurice the feet and wished him well.

chapter five

Immunosuppression and Academic Tenure

By the mid-1970s, we had largely convinced the cancer research community that FeLV caused leukemia as an infectious virus and that immunosurveillance sometimes worked effectively to prevent development of the cancer. The type of leukemia that most cats developed was lymphoblastic or lymphocytic, which might be diagnosed as either a blood leukemia or a solid tumor designated a lymphoma. But it was increasingly clear that other things were also going on after cats were infected with FeLV. Epidemiologically, the virus was also associated with a range of other diseases. Some were on the spectrum of hematological disorders like nonregenerative anemia or other types of leukemic or myeloproliferative diseases. It makes sense that both the lymphoid cancers and the anemias happened because FeLV had infected and transformed or altered some essential progenitor cells in bone marrow. But even beyond these diseases of blood and bone marrow, there was a clear epidemiologic association between FeLV and other serious opportunistic infections manifesting as pneumonias, peritonitis, and septicemias.[29] Some of these were lethal for cats before evidence of clinical leukemia was present. The only logical explanation was that the cats had an FeLV-induced immunosuppression.

Immunosuppression had been seen in people with rare genetic diseases like Wiskott-Aldrich syndrome or in people who were deliberately suppressed with drugs to allow organ transplantation. But prior to human acquired immunodeficiency syndrome (AIDS), immunosuppression had not been seen in people as the result of a viral infection. The pneumonias and septicemias of FeLV-infected cats seemed to have some of the same co-infections of bacteria, viruses, protozoa, or fungi that were later seen with human AIDS. These diseases might happen anyway in very old or debilitated cats. It was just that they happened much more often in young cats infected with FeLV.

It made sense that FeLV might also cause an AIDS-like disease because the target cell for the virus is thymus-derived lymphocytes, or T cells. While doing his autopsies on leukemic cats, Bill Jarrett had found that the thymus was seriously damaged and had evidence of extensive virus replication when examined with an electron microscope.[30] Another group at Ohio State University found that cats infected with FeLV were unable to reject skin grafts as would normal cats.[31] We also conducted a study to see if FeLV-infected cats could mount a typical vaccine-type antibody response, and we found that many could not.[32] Well before human AIDS had been seen, we had substantial evidence that a retrovirus, FeLV, could cause immune suppression.

Another disease often seen in FeLV-infected cats was glomerulonephritis, an inflammation of the kidneys. This is an immune complex type of disease that also occurs in people with systemic lupus erythematosus. So FeLV in cats is a multidimensional force in which the common theme is damage to the immune system. It could make immune cells cancerous and/or cause them to malfunction in various ways.

By now, most cancer researchers who were studying chicken or mouse retroviruses had given up on determining how or even whether those viruses caused cancer in free-living outbred species. They had, however, made progress in showing how some genes or proteins from those viruses could transform cultured cells to make them acquire properties that were characteristic of cancer cells.

Transformation of cells in the laboratory is thought to be an indication of what happens when normal cells become cancer cells in a person or animal. Radiation, certain chemicals, and some viruses, like retroviruses, can do this quite efficiently. One of the key properties expressed by both cancer cells and laboratory-cultured cells transformed by viruses is the ability of both to ignore signals to stop replicating. Normal cells, when cultured, will replicate in a petri dish or flask, but only to the point where the surface of the container is covered by a sheet of cells that are only a single layer thick. They will not keep growing by piling up, which is often called contact inhibition. The cultured cells will also exhibit senescence or aging after a number of replications that would be equivalent to the number seen in the normal aging process in a human or animal. Transformed cells, or cancer cells, on the other hand, will keep replicating. They may grow by piling up in a laboratory petri dish or by expanding beyond normal site limits or metastasizing in a person. They also show no aging and will continue to grow as long as nutrients are available. A good example of this is the so-called HeLa cell line. This source of immortal cancer cells was grown from a uterine cancer taken from Henrietta Lacks more than 70 years ago. Cultures of HeLa cells have been used for everything from studying cancer cell properties to growing numerous viruses ranging from polio to COVID. The history of this line of cultured cells was published as a popular book in 2010.[33]

Mouse and chicken retroviruses were shown to transform appropriate cells in culture and to cause solid tumors in animals if the replicating leukemia virus had incorporated an oncogene in the viral genome. When this happened, it sometimes made the oncogene-carrying virus unable to replicate, in which case it needed the leukemia virus to grow along with it as a helper virus. In some cases, the leukemia virus could incorporate the oncogene but still replicate effectively.

We conducted cell transformation with a feline sarcoma virus (FeSV), which may be present with the FeLV when the virus is found in cats with sarcoma-type solid tumors. When added to normal cell culture monolayers, this virus causes transformation. The transformed cells then contain a hybrid gene and its protein, which has both viral gene sequences and cellular oncogene sequences.[34] Ann Sliski, a PhD student in my group, conducted studies that showed that the transformed cells continued to replicate in the transformed phenotype even if the replicating FeLV disappeared, as long as the FeSV hybrid protein was still present.[35] This seemed important because it showed how a virus could make cells cancerous but no longer be present as a detectable virus. This provided at least a theoretical framework for how a virus could cause a cancer in a person by a "hit and run" mechanism where the virus brings in an oncogene that causes the transformation and disappears as a replicating virus by the time the cancer is diagnosed. Thus, failure to find a virus visually (that is, by electron microscopy) should not rule out the possibility that a virus could have initiated the process. We had also observed that the antibodies that mediated immunosurveillance-related regression of sarcomas in cats were directed to this hybrid protein composed partly of virus and partly of the oncogene product.

Overall, my research was going very well. I enjoyed teaching virology to graduate students and the intellectual stimulation that came from both students and other faculty. We were publishing frequently in the most competitive medical journals and had considerable outside interest in our results. I was invited to give lectures at numerous universities and at scientific meetings in places ranging from Venice and Amsterdam to Russia, Japan, and Argentina. I even received a few research awards, like the Bronze Medal from the American Cancer Society. While I thought that our research with FeLV was important for human cancer, I was still somewhat surprised when others seemed to agree.

One of the more interesting invitations I had was to be a visiting professor for a brief period at the University of Tehran. Neither Elizabeth nor I had been to the Middle East, so I accepted. Iran, particularly the Kurdish regions in the western part, were known for very high rates of esophageal cancer. The cause was unknown, and I was asked to consider the possibility of a virus. The invitation was from a former colleague from Iran who had returned home to build a center for immunology at the university. While there, I gave lectures in several places, and we were treated to a luxurious tour of the country. It included a stop at the Shah Abbas Hotel in Isfahan, then considered one of the most beautiful hotels in the world, and a visit to Shiraz and the ruins of Persepolis. It was just before the Islamic Revolution, which included the ouster of Shah Pahlavi and the occupation of the US Embassy with the taking of about 70 US citizens as hostages. The autocratic monarchy of the Shah had much internal opposition, including the academics. One day, all faculty, staff, and students at the university, including myself, were handed a rose and told they were required to go to a certain monument on campus and lay the rose to honor the birthday of the Shah's son. My Iranian friends were enthusiastic that the Shah might be forced out. But after it happened, they were surprised and depressed, not realizing that the government would soon become a theocracy under Supreme Leader Ayatollah Khomeini. Many academics and intellectuals then left the country, including our friend Farrokh, who moved to Geneva to work for the World Health Organization.

At Harvard, all junior faculty members are well aware of the "up or out" policy whereby new faculty have to be evaluated for promotion to full professor and academic tenure within 8 years of their first appointment. Promotion is based on excellence in teaching and research. However, winners of the Best Teacher Awards were often not promoted, while those with the largest research groups were almost always promoted. Teaching success is usually considered in a broad sense, beyond just classroom teaching, to include the mentoring of PhDs. Research success is based on the number and quality of publications and on competitive grant funding. Outside experts in the discipline of the candidate are always consulted during the review.

I had been promoted from assistant to associate professor in 1975. Most new faculty get this first promotion, but only a few reach the full professor level, which is customarily a lifetime appointment. Because of this, junior faculty at Harvard start to get anxious about their future after 5 or 6 years, and I was no different. To add to this, in the late 1970s there was a general awareness that President Bok had appointed our new dean, Howard Hiatt, to improve faculty quality at the school. Dean Hiatt, whom I respected, also seemed to be at odds about this with some of the senior faculty, including Dr. Nichols, who was my immediate supervisor as department chair.[24] Few, if any, junior faculty had been promoted to full professor with tenure from within the biomedical sciences since my arrival.

In this confusing environment, I felt I had to listen to some of the more interesting inquiries I received about potential positions outside Harvard. One of the most interesting, which I did explore, was at Washington State University (WSU) in Pullman. The dean and president there put together a very enticing package to appoint me as a professor and director of a new cancer research center. The benefits would include a new building to house my research, along with funding to recruit six new faculty in fields of my choosing. WSU and the state of Washington were interested in building a cancer research center at Pullman because they had had substantial success in building such a center earlier, the Fred Hutchinson Cancer Center in Seattle, at the other end of the state. It was recognized that cancer research was in a growth phase, and such an investment might stimulate academic research in the eastern part of the state. On one recruitment visit, I was hosted by the president of WSU and by Dr. Dixie Lee Ray, who was then the governor of Washington and a former head of the Atomic Energy Commission. It seemed like a big deal as we sat in the president's box at the University of Washington–WSU football game. I felt flattered and certainly had not been exposed to anything like this at Harvard. I decided to inquire among some of my junior colleagues to see if they would be interested in moving to WSU for a tenured professorship. Most said no. My wife, Elizabeth, who visited with me, was also unimpressed by the situation in Pullman.

As all of this was going on, our dean at the Harvard School of Public Health, Howard Hiatt, indicated that he really wanted me to stay in Boston and that I had a high likelihood of getting a tenured professorship soon. He consulted with my chair, Roger Nichols, who was much less enthusiastic. Dean Hiatt reminded Roger that department chairs were appointed by the dean, and Nichols soon resigned to become president of the Museum of Science in Boston.[24] A new ad hoc professorial committee was established to consider my promotion to full professor with tenure and to find a new department chair. It was a very impressive committee, having two Nobel laureates (Enders and Weller), the president of Memorial Sloan Kettering Cancer Center (Lewis Thomas), and the director of the Rockefeller Foundation (Ken Warren), along with several other professors from Harvard. The committee asked all senior faculty at the school to suggest candidates for the new chair's position. I suggested Bob Chanock, a flu expert at the NIH, and Peter Doherty, a veterinarian and immunologist from Australia who was also a Nobel laureate. After a few weeks, Dean Hiatt notified me that the committee had recommended me for a tenured professorship but with the condition that I also agree to serve as department chair. I wasn't very enthusiastic about being department chair but was greatly relieved to be offered the professorship. I then stayed as chair for 27 years and as a professor for 48 years. As chair, I soon realized that our most productive faculty seemed to prefer minimal supervision for their research and teaching. This seemed to work well for me also because it allowed me more time for my research. The long-term economic security provided by the tenure also allowed me to expand my research to look more directly at human cancer and immune suppression. The imminent discovery of the first human leukemia virus by a friend would present the opportunity to do so.

chapter six

Human Leukemia Virus

In the late 1960s and early 1970s, there were several reports of newly discovered human retroviruses postulated to be the causes of certain leukemias or lymphomas. All turned out to be false alarms or contaminants. Often they were xenotropic viruses of rodents, which only grow well when exposed, accidentally in this case, to cells from non-rodent species. It would usually be because human cancer cells were grown in labs where mouse cells were already present, and the endogenous xenotropic mouse virus would grow in the human cells. Many cancer researchers started to believe that human retroviruses would never be found, and derogatory terms like "human rumor viruses" came into vogue. The Special Virus Cancer Program of the National Cancer Institute (NCI) was gradually de-emphasized, but cancer research was still funded and encouraged for Nixon's "War on Cancer." Even if there were no retroviruses of humans, the leukemia viruses of cats, mice, and chickens could serve as molecular models for understanding the principles of how any causative agent might make a normal cell become a cancer cell and how that cancer cell could then grow uncontrolled in the body.

It was on this background that Dr. Robert Gallo, at the NCI, discovered the first RNA tumor virus or retrovirus that caused cancer in people. It was the end of the 1970s, and after nothing but false alarms, Gallo had trouble publishing his discovery.[36] But he persisted, and many papers were subsequently published after the first report in 1980.[37] The initial isolate, designated the human

T cell leukemia virus (HTLV), came from a man in the southeastern United States with an unusual form of T cell leukemia. As it turned out, leukemias of the same cell type were seen much more often in some other places. Dr. Kiyoshi Takatsuki, a pathologist from Kumamoto, had described a disease he called adult T cell leukemia (ATL) that seemed endemic in southwestern Japan.[38] It was a particularly aggressive cancer that was almost always fatal, with a usual survival time of just months after diagnosis. Japan is made up of four large islands. The disease was most common in the two southern islands, Kyushu and Shikoku, as well as in smaller islands like Okinawa, which were in the same region. When cases were found in more northern places in Japan, like Tokyo or Osaka, it was usually in people who were born and raised in the southern islands.

After Gallo's report of the HTLV, it was soon linked to ATL in Japan by Japanese investigators. They found that cases of ATL were almost always positive for infection with HTLV. Of even greater interest, perhaps, was that they also found that healthy adults in southern Japan were more likely to have antibodies to HTLV than healthy people either in the rest of Japan or in other countries. Healthy family members in the region who were living with someone who had ATL were even more likely to have antibodies to the virus. This obviously fit a pattern for a virus, in this case HTLV, that would be transmitted to those in closest contact. Further studies of antibody surveys suggested that the virus might be transmitted early in life, perhaps from mother to child, and also between spouses by sexual transmission.

As epidemiologists and other cancer researchers began to evaluate the importance of these results for other parts of the world, it soon became apparent that another high-risk area for HTLV and ATL already existed. This was the Caribbean basin, where places like Jamaica, Trinidad, and the northern coastal areas of Colombia and Venezuela also had elevated rates of ATL and HTLV antibodies. It is still unclear what these two areas of the world have in common, or conversely, why the virus and disease have not yet been found at higher rates in other major regions of the world that have been examined.

To make matters even more confusing, clinical epidemiologists soon found that HTLV was linked with another disease that seemed quite different from ATL. This disease was called tropical spastic paraparesis (TSP).[39] The most common symptom was lumbar backache and weakness in the legs that gradually progressed. TSP occurred primarily in the Caribbean basin and in southern Japan, the same places where HTLV occurred. Although both ATL and TSP were linked to HTLV, people got one or the other, not both. Among virologists, the question inevitably emerged of whether two different strains of HTLV might be involved in the two diseases, but no clear answer was forthcoming. Clinical neurologists also wondered whether HTLV might be a cause of multiple sclerosis (MS), which had overlapping symptoms with TSP, but patients with MS were not often infected with HTLV, and the geographic distribution of MS was clearly different from that of TSP and ATL.

Even before Gallo's discovery of HTLV, the US National Cancer Institute had a small budget that was specifically for small think tank workshops to be held periodically between Japanese and US scientists to discuss cancer research projects that were of particular interest to scientists from both countries. Presumably, the rationale was to form collaborations of mutual interest. Unlike most Asian countries, Japan already had a relatively large number of cancer researchers. In early 1982, Vince DeVita, then the director of the US National Cancer Institute, called for the workshop to take place in Seattle and to be focused on ATL and HTLV. The meeting had only 15 participants, with about half from each country. Gallo, who discovered HTLV, and Takatsuki, who first recognized ATL, were both there. I was invited to chair the meeting and to write a summary that would be published in a cancer research journal. Two scientists who were part of Gallo's team at the NCI were there. The other participants from the United States, including me, had never done research with HTLV or ATL, but all the participants from Japan, representing six different universities or cancer research institutes, were actively working with ATL and/or HTLV. The participants agreed that much progress had been made in the brief time since the first discoveries of the virus and the disease, and that research on the topic should be massively expanded to help us understand

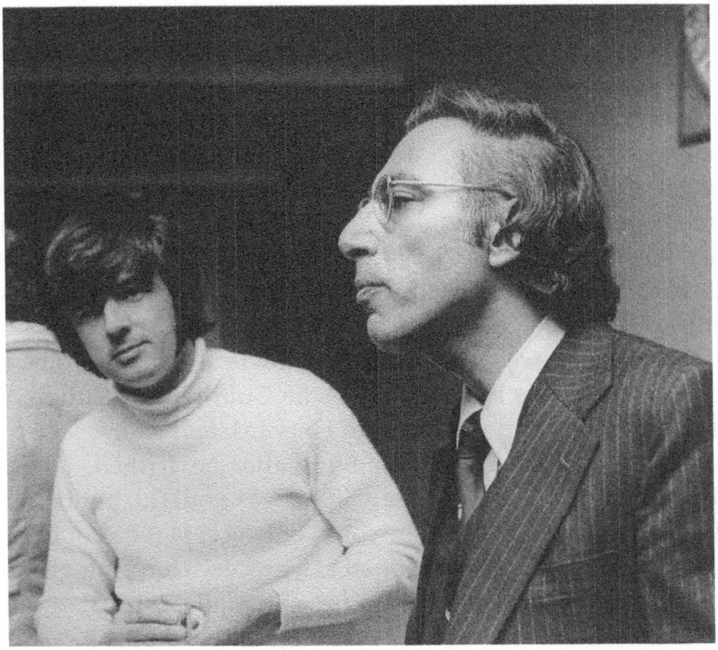

Figure 6.1: Max Essex, Bob Gallo

more about leukemia and how a virus could cause a human cancer. After the conclusion of the workshop, Bob Gallo asked me to stop for a drink at the hotel bar. We were alone, and the first words he said were, "Max, you have to start doing research on HTLV. As you see, there are many research projects to do, and a large number of Japanese researchers are working in this area, but almost nobody else is working on this in the US. I even have trouble getting some of the best people in my own lab to work on it, they've been so discouraged by the false alarms in the past about human tumor viruses. But this one is real. I'll give you all the reagents you need. We can do it by collaboration, or independently, that doesn't matter as long as we stay in communication." I thanked him and said I'd think about it. I was certainly just as convinced it was "real" as he was because I was so impressed about how FeLV caused cat leukemia. A few days after I got home, I called Gallo and said, "Bob, I'm in, send me the reagents."

My decision to get involved in HTLV research happened to coincide with a planned expansion of my research team to include several graduate students or junior scientists from Asia. The first three were from China but from rather different backgrounds. One was Dr. Zhu Shineng, a junior faculty pathologist from First Medical College in Shanghai. In the 1970s, there was an opening of relations between the People's Republic of China and the United States when Nixon and Henry Kissinger went to Beijing to meet with Mao. Sometimes called the "ping-pong" diplomacy, the two countries began to encourage cooperation in sports and academics. Zhu Shineng was one of the first medical scholars to be sent to the United States by China after the Cultural Revolution. Several of the first group were sent to Harvard, and Zhu selected my research group for his training. Soon after he arrived, Elizabeth and I invited him to dinner. He said he was grateful, but because I was his boss he insisted that he could only accept if he could make the dinner. We agreed. He stopped at a grocery store, bought some chicken, vegetables, and a few spices, and made a stir-fried dinner in our kitchen. He also insisted on doing the cleanup.

As part of the agreement between the United States and China, the mentor for each fellow, in this case me, would be invited to go to China to give a series of lectures following the return of the Chinese scholar. I did that and was moved by my experience in Shanghai. There were wide boulevards in China's largest city, but they were populated only with bicycles, not cars, and the people all wore blue or gray tunic uniforms. Zhu, an MD pathologist, told me his role during the Great Proletarian Cultural Revolution was to carry 50-pound bags of soil to establish new farms. I would go back to China quite a few times but usually not to Shanghai. When I did go back to Shanghai about three decades later, it seemed like the most modern and luxurious large city I had seen, with modern architecture and six-lane highways populated with luxury cars. Zhu then took me to dinner at the Four Seasons Hotel in his chauffeured car.

The other two new Chinese members of my lab group were from Taiwan. Both were recent graduates of National Taiwan University, which is the best college in the country, and both were accepted as doctoral student candidates at Harvard, after which they joined my research laboratory. Beyond that, their backgrounds were quite different. Ann-ping Chen was the daughter of the director of Veterans General Hospital, the largest academic hospital in Taiwan. Her family had come to the island of Taiwan following the revolution of Mao, when the previous Chinese government, under Chiang Kai-shek, settled in Taiwan to escape the communist revolution. Tun-Hou Lee, the other Taiwanese student who joined my lab, came from the smaller contingent of native Taiwanese who lived on the island before the arrival of the mainland Chinese. I was wary that the three Chinese students might not get along well with each other because of their very different backgrounds. I soon learned that there was no reason for such concern, as the three got along very well. After receiving her degree, Ann-ping returned to Taipei to become a faculty member at National Taiwan University. Tun-Hou, who did important research on HTLV for his doctoral thesis, did postdoctoral research in Stockholm at the same lab where I was trained and then returned to become a faculty member at Harvard. His research group then worked collaboratively with my own for decades, and our families became close friends. We still co-opt him for his bargaining skills whenever we buy a new car.

As our lab group got immersed in research on HTLV and ATL, I decided to focus on two issues right away. The first was whether HTLV might cause immunosuppression along with or in addition to causing leukemia. Almost all types of cancer have an associated risk for development of infectious diseases at their late terminal stage. But for FeLV-induced cat leukemia, where the virus infects T lymphocytes, as does HTLV, many cats develop immune suppression and serious problems with infectious diseases, even when they don't get the leukemia. We wondered if the same thing was true for people living in high-prevalence areas like southern Japan.

Through what seemed to be nothing more than a lucky break, a senior Japanese pathologist, Dr. Nobuyoshi Tachibana, wrote to see if I would accept him in my lab for a research sabbatical. He was based at the University of Miyazaki Medical School, which is one of the few cities in Kyushu, the southern island with the highest prevalence rate of HTLV. He was familiar with ATL and HTLV.

I eagerly accepted him and asked that he come as soon as possible and bring as many human samples as he could from HTLV-infected people. He arrived soon after, with a freezer box of human sera. We soon were able to set up a serology test to detect antibodies to HTLV using human cell lines and the same immunofluorescence protocols we had used to set up a test for FeLV antibodies in cats about 10 years before. We found that HTLV infection was also associated with immunosuppression-related infectious diseases in people, not just ATL. This obviously raised the related question of whether different variants of HTLV might be responsible for one type of pathology versus another in the cases of ATL, TSP, and immunosuppression.

While addressing the next question, concerning an accurate and sensitive test to better detect HTLV antibodies, we realized that it might be necessary to identify and characterize the viral surface protein so we could use it as the target for the antibodies. Some of the viral core antigens had already been identified and characterized, but they were less sensitive for detecting antibodies in people. The viral surface target of retroviruses is regularly a glycoprotein, or a protein linked to a sugar, which makes it harder to identify and purify.

Tun-Hou Lee, our brilliant laboratory tactician, had recently learned about a new technique called radiolabel sequencing, which seemed particularly appropriate for this problem. He went to the lab at the NIH that had perfected the technique for about a week, then came back to our lab to use it to identify the HTLV surface glycoprotein, called gp61.[40] After it became clear that widespread blood screening was needed to stop blood transfusion transmission of HTLV, our gp61 would be a necessary part of a test for blood safety. After noticing our results, the Harvard Patent Office submitted an application for the development of blood screening tests using gp61. The new technique was working so well that we also used it to search for the identity of the transforming protein that HTLV used to make normal lymphocytes become leukemic, and we soon found it.[41] A variation of this test is currently used for all blood collected for transfusion.

As we became more involved with research on human leukemia and HTLV, I was contacted by a veterinary pathologist at the New England Regional Primate Center, who said he had an outbreak of lymphoma at the facility and wondered if I was interested in looking at the monkeys. I said yes. We received samples and found that at least 11 of 13 monkeys with lymphoma had an HTLV-type virus based on the presence of antibodies.[42] The same antibodies were also present in about 7% of the healthy monkeys. This situation seemed remarkably similar to that of HTLV in the people of southern Japan. Macaques, the type of monkey involved in the New England Primate Center epidemic, are native to Asia, so we decided to try to get samples from Asian macaques and found that a similar number of them had antibodies to HTLV as well. This raised the obvious possibility that the leukemia epidemic in people in southern Japan might have started by the passage of HTLV or a related progenitor virus from macaque monkeys of the region to people. However, this could not explain why a similar epidemic was occurring in the Caribbean basin, as macaque monkeys are not present there.

The results of biomedical research inevitably lead to new questions and hypotheses. We were obviously motivated to study more about how different strains of HTLV and the monkey viruses could explain both the different diseases, like ATL versus TSP, and the distinct geographical patterns. Just about the time this was going on, however, I redirected much of our research program to a problem that was even more challenging – the new epidemic of immunosuppression in homosexual men that would later be called acquired immunodeficiency syndrome, or AIDS.

chapter seven

Cold Spring Harbor and the New Cancer Viruses

Cold Spring Harbor is a small village on the north shore of Long Island, about 40 miles from New York City. It is very well known to scientists for the Cold Spring Harbor Laboratory and Conference Center (CSH). The lab, though modest in size, has a reputation for outstanding research on cancer and genetics. The conference center has been the largest sponsor of research conferences on these topics for many decades. Almost all academic scientists in cancer research have been there for conferences; many would attend for a week or so every summer to present their own results and hear about progress from others on a particular topic, like retroviruses or cell biology.

The director of the Cold Spring Harbor Laboratory and Conference Center during the 1970s and 1980s was Dr. James Watson. He was sometimes referred to as the "father" of modern genetics because he, with Dr. Francis Crick, described the structure of DNA as a double helix.[43] For this, they won the Nobel Prize in 1962.

The late 1970s seemed like an appropriate time to take stock of the National Cancer Institute's Special Virus Cancer Program and Nixon's "War on Cancer" to see how well they were doing. One way to evaluate progress would be to look at advances in molecular genetics. There seemed to be no doubt that progress in this area had been immense. New tools that allowed one to look at how cancer cells go from normal to cancerous, how DNA may be repaired, and how single mutations in some cancers can be targeted for specific therapy were all becoming apparent. The new era of biotechnology for discovery of new pharmaceuticals, vaccines, and diagnostics was a direct result of government investment in research. Another way to look at progress, however, was to ask how much new evidence we had that viruses could cause naturally occurring cancers. Because much of the virus cancer research had been concentrated on retroviruses, and Gallo's discovery of HTLV had not been published until 1980, many were disappointed about the paucity of new knowledge about viruses causing human cancers. Soon, however, two major types of human cancer, those of the liver and the uterine cervix, would be linked to viruses. To address the issue, I was asked by Watson to help organize a conference on the topic at Cold Spring Harbor along with two friends as co-chairs. One was Dr. George Todaro, a senior scientist at the National Cancer Institute and an expert on how viruses make cells cancerous. Our lab had collaborated with his to study how the oncogene of the feline sarcoma virus could make cells cancerous. The other was Dr. Harald zur Hausen from Germany. Harald had done important work with herpes viruses, particularly the Epstein-Barr virus of Burkitt's lymphoma, and was now beginning to work on the possible role of papilloma viruses in human cancers. Some years later, I received the San Marino Prize jointly with zur Hausen for our research on viruses and cancer. Even later, he would win the Nobel Prize for his epic research proving that certain papilloma virus types were the cause of uterine cancer.[44] An effective vaccine is now available that can eliminate almost all risk of that disease.

The conference held at Cold Spring Harbor in 1980 had about 250 participants. The major conclusions would subsequently be published in a two-volume book.[45] The viruses covered included herpes, papilloma, and hepatitis B of people, along with many related and some unrelated viruses that cause cancer in chickens, mice, cats, cattle, and monkeys. The conference took place just before the first publication on the human T cell leukemia virus (HTLV), so it was too early for that topic to be included. About 4 years later, a separate CSH meeting and accompanying book on HTLV would be organized by Gallo, myself, and another old friend, Dr. Ludwik Gross.[46] Gross discovered the first murine leukemia virus, for which he received a Lasker Award, and published a major book on oncogenic viruses.[6] His daughter, Augusta, and her husband, Leslie, became family friends of Elizabeth and me.

Papilloma viruses occur in many species, where they cause benign growths in the skin, like warts. By the late 1970s, there was already evidence that papilloma viruses might also cause naturally occurring malignant tumors like carcinomas in rabbits and cattle. Probably, they cause benign and malignant tumors in other species as well, but research to verify this had not been done. The elegant research by zur Hausen showed not just that human papilloma virus (HPV) DNA was present in cells from cancers of the uterine cervix but that specific types of HPV, like types 16 and 18, were involved.[44] Very effective vaccines for HPV are now available and recommended for use before puberty for both girls and boys worldwide. The HPVs that are associated with cervix cancer are sexually transmitted. Although the vaccines are effective in the developing world as well, epidemiological evidence from several groups, including ours, suggests that the predominant types of HPVs in some regions of the world may be different from those of the United States and Europe.[47,48] More information is needed about possible differences in ratios of types that occur in developing countries. This seems important as the HPV-related diseases are most prevalent in Africa, Asia, and the Middle East. Additionally, it is increasingly clear that HPVs, especially type 16, which may be the most dangerous, are also associated with other types of mucosal malignancies. Existing HPV vaccines can prevent most of these.

Although cervix cancer could probably be eliminated with widespread use of the vaccine, some "anti-vaxxers" have interfered with the effectiveness of such public health programs. Some question the vaccine's safety or efficacy, and some argue that its use might increase sexual promiscuity.[49] These and some other groups resist the use of the vaccine in boys, presumably because they don't get cervix cancer. They do, however, transmit the virus and can develop certain cancers of the oropharyngeal and anogenital areas.[50]

Until the late 1970s, many scientists thought that herpesviruses, like herpes simplex that causes genital and oral ulcers, might be the cause of cervix cancer. That didn't pan out. Herpes viruses like the Epstein-Barr virus (EBV) are still important as a cause of Burkitt's lymphoma (BL) and nasopharyngeal carcinoma. These cancers were rare until the AIDS epidemic, but BL became much more common in people suffering from immunosuppression caused by human immunodeficiency virus (HIV). Another rare type of cancer that is common in AIDS patients is Kaposi sarcoma (KS). KS is a cancer of blood vessels that emerges as red or purple spots on the skin but also in many internal sites that are not readily visible. KS is caused by a herpesvirus designated the human herpesvirus 8 (HHV8) or the Kaposi sarcoma–associated herpesvirus (KSHV).[51] It appears to be sexually transmitted and present in many people, while only causing KS in people who are immunosuppressed, such as by HIV. KS is also a very unusual type of cancer as it is polyclonal. Most forms of cancer are monoclonal, arising from a single transformed cell, regardless of whether that original cancer cell was made malignant by a virus, irradiation, or a chemical carcinogen.

One of the most important types of cancer caused by a virus is primary liver cancer, or hepatoma. It is caused primarily by hepatitis B virus, though another virus, hepatitis C virus, can also be involved. Hepatitis B virus (HBV) particles, also called Dane particles, have a DNA genome like papilloma viruses or herpes viruses, unlike retroviruses like FeLV or HTLV, which have RNA genomes. Remarkably, HBV still replicates by going through an RNA stage using reverse transcriptase as would a retrovirus.

HBV was first linked to liver cancer through a large seroepidemiology project conducted by Dr. R. Palmer Beasley in Taiwan. Even in the 1970s, Taiwan had very good health records and blood samples from all the national employees. Palmer checked blood samples from more than 22,000 employees and showed that those who were viremic with HBV, or had Dane particles, had a 60-fold increased risk for the development of liver cancer. For this work, he received the General Motors Prize. While I was at a virus conference with Palmer in Riyadh, Saudi Arabia, we were asked by the World Health Organization (WHO) to meet with the Saudi health minister to convince him to use the HBV vaccine more widely in the kingdom. We thought he had reservations about the safety or efficacy of the vaccine, as it was relatively new. He listened to our message and had a simple reply. He said he had no concerns about the safety of the vaccine but thought the cost, which was then about $100 per dose, was too high. He said the country would purchase the vaccine, and vaccinate all, if the cost were reduced. The price of the vaccine was reduced, and it soon became widely used in Saudi Arabia.

My first serious introduction to hepatitis B research came in Dakar, Senegal, when I was invited to a small meeting by Dr. Philippe Maupas, a professor at the University of Tours in France. Philippe was unusual in that he had three earned doctoral degrees – one an MD, another in veterinary medicine, and a PhD in microbiology. He was the first to make an HBV vaccine, and I, along with several others at the meeting, were among the first human subject volunteers to be injected with it. That first batch was made from Dane particles concentrated from infected people. The HBV would have been killed, but some of the donors apparently had bacterial infections as several of us who were newly vaccinated got fever, presumably from an endotoxin. I felt lucky as I did not have any side effects, and all of us had good antibody responses to HBV.

Philippe and I became quick friends and discussed research collaboration on several aspects of HBV infection. Things then took a tragic turn when Philippe was killed in a car crash soon after. He had just flown from Senegal to Paris on a late flight and apparently fell asleep while driving from Paris to his home in Tours. We were devastated, but a group of younger students and fellows in his research group carried on the work. Four of them joined my lab in Boston to continue some of the experiments we planned. One, Dr. Jean-Loup Romet-Lemonne, did important research to show that HBV replicated in the bone marrow of carriers, as well as in the liver, which helped to explain how the infectious disease could remain latent for long periods at the incubation period before disease develops.[52] Another, Camille Sureau, had the first successful replication of HBV in cells cultured in a laboratory. He used closed circles of HBV DNA, which was transduced, as naked DNA, into liver cells, achieving the first laboratory production of Dane particles.[53] Even back to the days of polio, the development of techniques to produce infectious virus in laboratory cell cultures has often been an important step for subsequent work to make drugs, diagnostics, and vaccines. The third fellow who came to me from Maupas was Dr. Philippe Roingeard. Philippe extended some of the work of Camille by characterizing the HBV that was produced in laboratory cultures. He also did some important seroepidemiological studies with our collaborators, showing that perinatal infections were common in infants born to HBV-infected nursing mothers.[54]

The fourth person who joined our group from the Maupas lab was Dr. Francis Barin. Francis switched to work with HIV and made great strides on development of tests for diagnosing HIV infections. He returned to France and became a professor at the University of Tours. We also became great friends, and Holly, our oldest daughter, got to spend a summer living with his family in France while trying to learn French.

In the early years, HBV was thought of as a virus that was transmitted primarily by blood transfusion, especially by the researchers and medical experts who focused their studies on the United States and Europe. But then, researchers focused on Africa and Asia realized that the highest rates of infection occurred in African and Asian countries where blood transfusions were rare. In the United States, the highest rates were in homosexual men, even before the development of the AIDS epidemic. Subsequent studies showed infectious HBV in vaginal fluids, saliva, semen, and breast milk, with the highest rates found in places with poor socioeconomic conditions. More than half of the infants born to viremic mothers get lifelong infections. Clustering occurs in families, but it is primarily due to HBV exposure and transmission, not genetics. It has been estimated that more than 300 million people are lifelong carriers. They live primarily in Africa and Asia, where up to 10% of the population may be infected. In Europe and the United States, only about 0.1% of the population are infected. As with HPV and cervix cancer, the developing world has the largest burden of disease. We have very good vaccines to prevent both major cancers, and it is a sad commentary on health and human rights that the populations who need these vaccines the most have the least access to them.

Dane particles, which turned out to be infectious HBV, were first identified in the blood of an Aboriginal Australian by Dr. Barry Blumberg in 1966. For this, he received the Nobel Prize in 1975. Sharing the prize with him was Dr. Carleton Gajdusek, whom I knew fairly well. Carleton received the prize for his research on kuru, showing that the cause was a "slow virus," or prion. Kuru is a neurological disease that occurred primarily in New Guinea, where transmission occurred through cannibalism, when the New Fore people would eat the brains of their dead ancestors to gain knowledge. Carleton was very bright and spoke many languages. He lived among the New Fore people for years and learned their language, allowing him to trace the disease cases to the practice of ritualistic cannibalism.

I recall discussing the case of Gajdusek with Dr. Stanley Prusiner in London at a dinner at the home of Marguerite Littman, who was a major supporter of AIDS causes in Great Britain. Stanley later received the Nobel Prize for his characterization of the prion infectious agent of scrapie in sheep. The causative agents of scrapie and kuru are related to the agent of "mad cow" disease, which occurs in cattle when they eat the flesh or bones of other cattle who had the disease in reprocessed cattle food. Mad cow disease can also be transmitted to people who eat beef, though this disease in people, where it is called Creutzfeldt-Jakob disease, has been largely eliminated as of 2010 or 2015. Following a modest epidemic about 20 years ago, many Europeans stopped eating beef. British Airways, for example, replaced beef on their menus with ostrich steaks.

Scrapie and kuru are neurological diseases, not cancers, and the "slow viruses" that cause these diseases are usually unrelated to the known classes of human cancer viruses. However, the epidemiology of virus-related neurological diseases may pose similar challenges to that of virus-caused cancers. Surprisingly, the first human retrovirus discovered was soon shown to be linked to both an unusual leukemia and an unusual neurological disease.[39]

In conclusion, some viruses, like COVID, cause disease by a very straightforward transmission pattern, making them easy to trace. Others, like the viruses that cause cancer, immunosuppression, or some neurological diseases, are much harder for epidemiologists to unravel. The next new epidemic, AIDS, would challenge us even more before new scientific knowledge and political responses could provide help.

chapter eight

AIDS: The Beginning

The first recognition of the disease we now call AIDS was in the summer of 1981. Dr. Myron Gottlieb, a physician at the University of California at Los Angeles (UCLA) Medical School, described five cases of Pneumocystis pneumonia in homosexual men.[55] Pneumocystis pneumonia had been seen before but usually only in severely debilitated cancer patients who had been on unsuccessful chemotherapy and were near death. The new cases were young men who were healthy until their recent rapid deterioration, and they had no other apparent malignancy or chemotherapy. Soon after, many other cases were reported, especially in San Francisco and New York City, and in sections of those cities where men who had sex with men were more likely to reside. In retrospect, other clinicians also mentioned seeing occasional cases prior to 1981, even in the late 1970s, but since they were isolated, they were not mentioned to public health officials or described in print. Pneumocystis is a fungus that is ubiquitous in the lungs of many species, but it almost never causes disease except in people with severe immunosuppression. The drug used to treat the disease, pentamidine, was not generally available. When oncologists needed it, they contacted the Centers for Disease Control and Prevention (CDC), who had a supply. In late 1981 and 1982, the CDC noticed that requests for the drug were rapidly increasing.

When Gottlieb published his paper in the *New England Journal of Medicine*, the CDC immediately sensed something new and published an alert for the medical and public health community in their *Morbidity and Mortality Weekly Report*. At about the same time, or soon after, the medical community recognized what appeared to be an accompanying epidemic of Kaposi sarcoma in the same populations of homosexual men. Until then, Kaposi sarcoma was also virtually unknown to occur in young Caucasian men, though it was occasionally seen in elderly Mediterranean men and in people from sub-Saharan Africa. The cause of Kaposi, human herpesvirus 8, is now known, but it wasn't known then. Other reports of unusual diseases in men who had sex with men would also be reported soon after. These included a form of tuberculosis caused by Mycobacterium avium, a pathogen of birds; cryptococcal meningitis; and toxoplasmosis. All of these diseases were known to exist but usually only in debilitated end-stage cancer patients.

The only logical explanation for this constellation of outcomes was that the patients had an underlying destruction of their immune system. Gottlieb had an astute observation that verified this: the ratio of T helper and T suppressor immune lymphocytes was imbalanced. The ratio usually seen in healthy adults is about 2:1, two helper cells for each suppressor cell. The ratio in these patients was more like 0.2:1. Studies by clinical immunologists soon showed that the real problem was a reduction or loss of T helper cells, which are needed to activate the immune system. In end-stage patients with Pneumocystis, the T helper cells were greatly reduced or totally gone. The new disease was then called gay-related immunosuppressive disease, or GRID.

Almost as soon as the term GRID was suggested, it appeared to be incomplete or incompatible with the new disease, as cases of the same type of immune suppression were seen in other groups of people as well. The first was injection drug users (IDUs), who had the same lethal outcomes and a lack of immune helper T cells. In some places, like Newark, New Jersey, the number of cases in IDUs was as high or higher than the number of cases in men who had sex with men. A new definition of community-acquired immunodeficiency disease, or CAIDS, was then proposed.

The next group to experience the same disease was hemophiliacs. Until the early 1980s, many hemophiliacs often needed blood transfusions. But at about the same time that AIDS started, the purified clotting factor VIII became available. However, factor VIII was made from concentrated blood pooled from hundreds or thousands of donors. The new name of CAIDS seemed to need to drop the C, as hemophiliacs don't necessarily live in communities. So it became just AIDS. Then AIDS was seen in some blood transfusion recipients (who presumably got the disease in the same way as hemophiliacs or IDUs) who might have been exposed to bad blood as "mini-transfusions" on contaminated needles that were passed around. A similar AIDS-like disease was then seen in some people of Haitian origin, which seemed like an entirely different risk group. Rumors then circulated that they might be in the loop if gay men were frequenting Haiti for sex tourism. It was also mentioned that some batches of clotting factor VIII for hemophiliacs were made from blood collected from paid donors in Haiti. Vulgar comments about avoiding the "4-H club" (homosexuals, heroin users, hemophiliacs, Haitians) sometimes surfaced from the demagogues.

Patients who developed AIDS often had enlarged lymph nodes or lymphadenopathy before they developed the end-stage diseases like Pneumocystis pneumonia. Candidiasis or thrush was also common at the early stages. More blood transfusion recipients were found with the disease as well as some women and infants. Most of the women were IDUs themselves or partners of bisexual men or IDUs. The infected infants were usually found to be born to women who were either IDUs or recipients of transfusions.

The US Centers for Disease Control and Prevention (CDC) mobilized an epidemiology task force to investigate the outbreak soon after the first cases were reported in gay men. The CDC is the federal agency that normally looks into reports of new or unusual diseases. They have a good track record for the rapid determination of the cause of outbreaks like Legionnaires disease, Ebola, or gastroenteritis on cruise ships. But AIDS was completely different. Although gay men were an obvious risk group, it was not at all clear that each case was connected to another case. Extensive questionnaires and interviews were used to determine that gay men who developed AIDS were more likely to have more partners, anonymous partners, and receptive anal sex without condoms.

One airline steward, Gaetan Dugas, proudly proclaimed to have had thousands of recent sex partners.[56] It seemed possible that some people like him were "Typhoid Marys" or hypertransmitters, but that wasn't enough to explain all the peculiarities of how the disease was transmitted.

In the early 1980s, most epidemiologists, including those at the CDC, followed protocols for contact tracing, seeking cases that were linked in time and place. This did not work very well if the disease took a long and variable time to develop, or if the cases were likely to transmit long before they developed disease, or if many who were exposed to the same risk factors did not develop the disease at all. And the CDC had a very limited budget to investigate new diseases. Most of their budget was limited to the routine collection of morbidity and mortality data. As the numbers of reported cases rapidly increased, more clinicians and epidemiologists began to study the disease in a multidisciplinary manner, especially in the cities with the largest number of cases.

Several months after the first reports of AIDS, the US NIH hosted a think tank–type workshop to discuss possible theories about what the cause might be. There seemed to be good agreement that the disease was an acquired immunodeficiency characterized by the severe reduction or loss of T helper cells (T helper cells were also called T4 cells because of a common reagent used to count their number). Several of the epidemiologists present had focused on behavioral issues. One group proposed that the cause might be the amyl and butyl nitrate "poppers" that were used by some gay men to enhance sexual performance. Another group of immunologists proposed that receptive rectal sex with semen deposition might cause an autoimmune type of reaction. The third group, and certainly the one to which I belonged, proposed that an infectious agent, especially a virus, might be the cause. Among the advocates for a viral cause were several herpes experts. Herpes simplex was known to be sexually transmitted. The Epstein-Barr herpes virus was known to be the cause of Burkitt's lymphoma, although it was a disease of B lymphocytes, not T lymphocytes. Kaposi sarcoma, which was common in AIDS patients, was thought to be associated with a herpes virus, though the true identity of that virus wouldn't be known until the 1990s.[18] Some proposed a role for hepatitis B virus (HBV), which was known to be sexually transmitted and more prevalent in homosexual men. It was not known to infect lymphocytes, but about 2 years later, our lab showed that it could (see chapter 6).

Bob Gallo and I were at the meeting, and we hypothesized that a human retrovirus might be a cause of AIDS. The T cell lymphotropic virus of cats caused both leukemia and immunosuppression, as did the human T cell leukemia virus (HTLV) (see chapters 5 and 6). HTLV also caused the neurological disease tropical spastic paraparesis. If that was due to a separate strain of HTLV, perhaps AIDS might be due to another variant of the virus. For the next year or two, Gallo and I talked often about our hypothesis, plans, and later, results. To avoid interruptions, we spoke by phone most Saturdays for an hour or more. The CDC also seemed to be leaning toward an infectious origin for AIDS. Dr. Don Francis, a member of their task force, had done his research training in my lab. His doctoral thesis in 1979 was on transmission of the feline leukemia virus, and he left very impressed with how the virus caused immunosuppression in cats. His assignment upon returning to CDC would be to work with hepatitis B virus. By the time AIDS was recognized a few years later, his usual comment would be, "This disease looks like a combination of feline leukemia and hepatitis B." His CDC colleagues were probably not so impressed, thinking these two viruses were the only two that Don had studied in any detail.

At the same time, the CDC did not seem to be very aware of the HTLV that had recently been discovered by Gallo. By 1981 or 1982, confirmation of Gallo's discovery had been published by Japanese investigators, and much new information was being revealed. The CDC published an extensive study comparing infection rates or seroprevalence for more than 20 infectious agents in AIDS patients versus controls. Most common bacterial and viral infections known to be sexually transmitted were included, but HTLV was not.[57] None of the microbes studied stood out as likely to be linked to AIDS.

Gay activists were becoming very involved, warning men who had sex with men about having multiple sex partners and harassing politicians like Ed Koch, the mayor of New York City, to do more on prevention. Larry Kramer, a playwright in New York whom I would later get to know, had tremendous impact. He started the Gay Men's Health Crisis Center and ACT UP (AIDS Coalition to Unleash Power). These and other derivative organizations made a huge difference educating both at-risk gay men and community and political leaders who just wanted to avoid the issue. With his play *The Normal Heart* and book *Faggots*, he also had substantial outreach to educate some who came from outside the gay community. Cleve Jones was an independent leader and educator for the gay community in California, but neither he nor anyone else was sufficiently influential to stop the high-risk lifestyle epitomized by the bathhouses. Later, Cleve would go on to develop the Quilt Project, which tried to include a panel in the name of each person who died of AIDS. Eventually, it would become the largest piece of folk art in the world, with more than 50,000 panels. The quilt began to increase awareness of the devastation as it grew, even educating many outside the gay community. Randy Shilts, a gay reporter for the *San Francisco Chronicle*, was one of the first journalists to write extensively about AIDS for the mainstream press. He would later publish a diary type of book about his observations during the early stages of the epidemic.[56] The book, *And the Band Played On*, was also made into a movie. The movie depicted Gallo as an antihero, which was totally inaccurate, and the actor who played me was bald. My full head of hair may be my best feature. Shilts died of AIDS in 1994.

Convincing gay men at high risk to change their lifestyle was huge, but getting others like politicians and scientists to help solve the problem was just as difficult. The mayors of New York and San Francisco, the cities most affected, were Ed Koch and Dianne Feinstein. Even though both were from a liberal Democratic background, they were reluctant to get involved with either public messaging or funding. Most politicians avoided talking about AIDS. Tim Westmoreland, a senior aide to California Congressman Henry Waxman, seemed to be the only one who wanted the federal government to get involved. President Reagan totally ignored the problem, gaining deserved damnation for refusing to use the word

"AIDS." Some religious zealots claimed AIDS was God's curse on homosexuals. The Moral Majority under Jerry Falwell acted in an immoral way and counseled the federal government to stay away from the problem. Pat Buchanan, a perennial right-wing presidential candidate who also preceded Tucker Carlson on CNN's *Crossfire*, stoked fear against gay physicians and gay men employed in schools, restaurants, and hotels.

Shilts and the CDC also expressed frustration about the reluctance of scientists to find the cause and help solve the problem. This was true but in part because of a lack of financial support to do the research. Most laboratory research is very expensive, and almost all research is done through competitive grants from the NIH or other national agencies. The grants must be applied for 6–12 months in advance, and funds are awarded for very specific projects. Grant funds awarded for the study of ovarian cancer or spinal cord injuries cannot be used to study AIDS. To overcome this, several programs began to raise money to award small grants, but the establishment of the programs took time, and the funding that became available was usually too small to attract the A-list scientists.

Most of the physicians who became involved in AIDS came from a background of specialization in either infectious diseases or oncology. Infectious disease specialists are often called in to treat end-stage infections like Pneumocystis or cryptococcal meningitis in cancer patients. Oncologists were brought in to treat Kaposi sarcoma and the lymphomas that occur in AIDS patients. Most oncologists and infectious disease doctors on the front lines in large city clinics are not themselves involved in lab research and probably have little or no time away from their clinical duties to communicate with the mainstream researchers. Some clinicians devoted much of their attention to AIDS cases. Those responsible for blood banks were one of the groups of medical professionals who felt distressed and highly motivated.

Quite apart from AIDS, the government soon realized that the medical research community needed more physician-scientists and offered financial support to Harvard and many other medical centers to train more researchers. Major changes were also underway in the training of epidemiologists. During the 1970s, many academic epidemiologists stopped studying infectious diseases, thinking such problems had been solved. Most were now studying chronic diseases like cancer or cardiovascular problems. Understanding the cause of AIDS would require more of a multidisciplinary approach than most other diseases.

Only a few lab scientists were getting involved. Most, like my group, were virologists. Except for Dr. Tony Fauci, most immunologists seemed uninterested. By 1982, hundreds of documented cases were reported by the CDC. We decided to give it our best effort to seek the cause of AIDS.

chapter nine

Finding the Cause

Mobilizing laboratory researchers to get involved in the AIDS problem was also difficult. Some scientists were reluctant to get involved for fear of infecting themselves or their colleagues. When our lab staff first got involved at Harvard, some fearful neighbors in the department put epoxy glue in our lab door locks to try to prevent our work, and a few clerical staff threatened to quit, even though they were not permitted to go into the lab. We tried to devise ways to get samples to the lab so people wouldn't be unnecessarily afraid. There were many examples of the fear of AIDS that developed in the general public.

Ryan White was an Indiana boy with hemophilia who developed AIDS in 1984 from the weekly infusions of factor VIII that he needed to allow normal blood clotting. Because of widespread fear and ignorance about AIDS, he was blocked from attending school by teachers and the parents of other students. When he was later permitted to go to school, half of the other students stayed home. He soon became a poster child for the AIDS epidemic. A movie was made about his life. Much later, when the government would finally provide federal funding for people with AIDS, the legislation was called the Ryan White Care Act. In Florida, a family with three hemophiliac boys were exiled from their community, and their house was burned down. The fear was depressing and irrational, but real. We now think of homophobia as almost synonymous with bigotry against homosexuals. But in the 1980s, it was more than that. It was also associated with the fear of catching AIDS, especially if the cause was a new and mysterious virus.

When a new disease is seen in people, it is usually either because of transmission from an animal reservoir or because of an important genetic mutation in an existing microbe. In many cases, it is both: a mutation or set of mutations in an animal virus that makes it more transmissible and more likely to be able to expand its host range. A given virus may have evolved to grow best in bats or mice or monkeys by virtue of its surface protein forming a bond with a receptor on the host cell surface. The host cell receptor may be specific to mucosal cells lining the nasal and pharyngeal passages of the upper respiratory tract, or it may be specific to the digestive tract or the reproductive organs. Many viruses also then replicate in the blood as a viremia. Only a few mutations, or sometimes even one mutation, can make a virus surface protein better able to attach to, and thus enter, a wider variety of cells. This type of mutational change may make a virus more able to infect additional types of cells, like lung cells, rather than just pharyngeal cells. If so, a virus that only caused a common cold or pharyngitis may now also cause pneumonia. Or another mutational change in the viral surface protein that previously made it attach only to monkey cells might now allow the virus to also attach to human cells.

Viruses that have RNA genomes usually make the most errors when they copy their genes, and thus they are the fastest to accumulate more mutations. Coronaviruses like COVID and retroviruses are both RNA viruses with high mutation rates. Flu is as well, but it also has an additional method of changing its surface proteins and thus its transmission properties. Flu genomes have separate pieces of RNA for each gene. When a single host cell is infected by two different flu viruses, reassortment of the genes results in the progeny viruses becoming hybrids and immediately acquiring some of the characteristics of both parental viruses. Many public health experts are worried about a flu virus that is currently causing a serious epidemic in birds moving to people where it might cause a pandemic that is even worse than the COVID pandemic.

When AIDS was first recognized, it was particularly difficult to understand because it didn't fit the pattern of any previous epidemic, like flu or a gastroenteritis. AIDS was Kaposi sarcoma in one person, pneumonia in another, and encephalitis in a third for an almost endless number of signs and symptoms. For most new epidemics, the respiratory or gastrointestinal disease occurs only a few days or a week after the newly infected person had contact with the previous case. For AIDS, most people showed no serious signs or symptoms until months or years after exposure to the last case, even though most people would die from the infection, at least until the 1990s when good combinations of drugs were available to prevent disease progression and death. This extreme variation in signs and symptoms as well as the prolonged time to disease development obviously made it very difficult to do contact tracing as a way to identify a common cause.

Most virologists specialize. Although they would normally teach about all viruses in the classroom, for their research they would normally focus on just one virus or perhaps a phylogenetic group of viruses, like herpes or retroviruses. In 1982, only two viruses were known to infect lymphocytes. One was the Epstein-Barr virus, which only infected B lymphocytes. The other was HTLV, which specifically infects T lymphocytes. As AIDS was better characterized by pathologists, it became clear that the disease was immunosuppression due to a loss of T lymphocytes. As HTLV was only recently discovered, only a few lab groups had the expertise and the reagents to work with it. One was Gallo's group, as they discovered the virus, and another was our lab. So by 1982, both of our groups hypothesized that an HTLV-related retrovirus could be the cause of AIDS, and we began laboratory experiments to test the hypothesis.

The next challenge for our lab group was to get adequate numbers of blood samples, or at least blood plasma samples, from well characterized AIDS patients and suitable uninfected control subjects. Even then, it was unclear what the best control group might be. As it seemed to take many months to develop clinical AIDS, it seemed possible or even likely that some of the control subjects from the same risk groups, like gay men or injection drug users, might themselves already be positive for the putative causative agent. If the causative agent caused disease in some but not all, perhaps some healthy contact subjects would already have antibodies to the new virus. By the fall of 1982, we did get samples from the US CDC. The CDC, which had the largest number of well characterized samples, sent us a large batch in late 1982. They were matched with a similarly large number of controls of various types, all of which were sent under code. We also received some AIDS patient samples from Dr. Martin Hirsch, the head of viral diseases at Massachusetts General Hospital and a friend.

In the May 20, 1983, issue of *Science* magazine, there were five publications on AIDS, the first to provide experimental data on a possible cause. The first two were from my group,[32,58] the next two were from Gallo's group,[59,60] and the fifth was from the Luc Montagnier group at the Pasteur Institute in Paris, France.[61] Our first paper was just about cats, showing that FeLV-infected cats had severe suppression of their antibody responses, providing good evidence for why they developed AIDS-like disease.

Our second paper was on human AIDS, utilizing the sera from the CDC-characterized AIDS patients. They were tested for antibodies to HTLV producer lymphocytes using membrane immunofluorescence of living cells, the same test we used to detect antibodies in Japanese T cell leukemia patients.[62] We found that 25% of 75 AIDS patients with Kaposi sarcoma or Pneumocystis pneumonia were positive, as were 26% of 23 patients with pre-AIDS or lymphadenopathy syndrome. One of 81 matched healthy homosexual male controls was positive. Only 1 of 305 other control samples was positive, including unmatched homosexual men, blood donors, kidney dialysis patients, and hepatitis patients. This was the first evidence, along with the accompanying papers from the Gallo and Montagnier groups, that a retrovirus was associated with AIDS.

The first of two papers from Gallo's group used DNA hybridization to look for HTLV-related gene sequences in cells from AIDS patients. Two of 33 were positive. The second paper described the isolation and growth of HTLV from one AIDS patient in cell culture and the finding of HTLV-related proteins in two more AIDS patients. The paper from Montagnier's lab describes a retrovirus isolated from a homosexual patient with pre-AIDS lymphadenopathy. That paper describes the virus as "a member of the human T cell leukemia virus family" and states that the serum from the AIDS patient "reacted strongly with antigens on the surface of HTLV-infected cells."

Collectively, these papers provided a clear lead – that something related to HTLV was going on with at least some of the AIDS patients. But because the Gallo and Montagnier papers were only on one or two selected patients, and our seroepidemiology study showed only a quarter to a third of AIDS patients to be positive, there was certainly not proof of cause.

The fact that these papers were about to be published was somehow leaked to the press. The normal procedure would be that *Science* magazine would inform the press about new research to be published about a week before the actual publication date. The day before the press was to be informed, I was returning home from a consultation with Gallo and others at the National Cancer Institute. Starting at about 9 pm, I received calls from several medical journalists from the *Boston Globe*, the *New York Times*, and other major newspapers. After feeling harassed and awkward about refusing to comment before the *Science*-imposed embargo when the first journalists called, I told my oldest daughter, Holly, that she could stay on the phone for an hour or more talking to her friends. As a young teenager, she was always eager to spend more time on the phone. We had only one line, and no cell phones yet, so this would hopefully dissuade the reporters after they got a busy signal. It was probably bad judgment on my part as some of them persisted, thinking the phone was tied up because I was talking to other reporters. One national nightly news program showed a photo of the Harvard building where my lab was based with a comment that they knew there was some new information from my lab and from Gallo's, but we wouldn't tell them what it was. The next day, the embargo was lifted, we were instructed to talk to the press, and we did our best to put the findings in perspective.

The lead journalist from the *Boston Globe* who was upset with me for not talking sooner was Loretta McLaughlin. She became a strong voice in support of research and governmental responsibility for AIDS support. Through her position as editor of the editorial page of the *Boston Globe*, that newspaper became a leader for educating the public about AIDS. Loretta got her start as an investigative journalist who uncovered the crime spree of the "Boston Strangler." After her retirement, she devoted her services to the Harvard AIDS Institute as a writer.

As soon as we finished the study published in the May 20, 1983, issue of *Science*, we began a new study to look for HTLV-related antibodies in hemophiliacs. Using the same criteria as we described in the earlier study, two of three cases of hemophiliacs with AIDS were positive for HTLV-related antibodies, as were 7% of asymptomatic hemophiliacs.[63] Only 1 of 234 controls, including blood donors, healthy lab workers, dialysis patients, and hepatitis patients, was positive. This extended the concern that hemophiliacs had an elevated risk for exposure to an HTLV-related virus, but we had too few cases of hemophiliac AIDS to shed new light on actual cause. *Science* magazine was obviously very interested in the issue, as they published the paper less than a month after it was submitted. This is extraordinarily rapid, normally only done in cases of national emergency.

Just 6 months later, our lab published another paper in *Science*. It was on how transfusion-associated cases of AIDS could be linked to an HTLV-positive blood donor. It was again published less than a month after submission.[64] This study was also done in collaboration with the CDC. Dr. Harold Jaffe there had carefully collected blood samples from 12 patients with transfusion-associated AIDS. Samples were only available for 8 of the AIDS patients, and 3 were positive. Samples were only available from 117 of the 157 donors, but 9 were positive. Of particular interest, an HTLV antibody–positive donor was identified for 6 of the 12 transfusion-associated AIDS cases. Of unrelated blood donors, only 1 of 298 was positive. Statistically, it was determined that this association of transfusion-AIDS donors with HTLV-related antibodies would only occur once in 10,000 instances if due to chance alone. While highly significant, this still did not explain why a larger fraction of AIDS patients were not positive for the antibodies.

At the same time all this was going on, molecular biologists at Harvard and many other research-rich institutions were being encouraged to help industry develop their inventions so they would be available for application in the health-care system more rapidly. Harvard had a newly energized Patent Office that would proactively meet with selected faculty to review discoveries for possible submission of relevant patent applications. After a review of our work, which was sure to attract their attention because of the press coverage, the Harvard Patent Office took responsibility for drafting patent protection for several of the HTLV antigens. We had just finished identifying and characterizing the viral surface protein that was most valuable for blood screening.[65] They projected that it would now be necessary to screen blood for HTLV, regardless of whether or not it was a cause of AIDS. It was already clear that it was contaminating the blood supply, and tests were needed to assure blood safety.

Along with the push for patents, Harvard set up new guidelines whereby faculty would be encouraged to get involved in corporate research programs. At the School of Public Health, faculty would be allowed to consult for pharmaceutical or biotechnology companies for up to 1 day per week. In return, faculty could receive financial compensation or company stock shares for their effort. The Harvard Medical School even had a pool of money that would be available for new Harvard-linked biotechnology companies to allow closer monitoring of such activities.

Dr. William Haseltine was one of the brightest molecular biologists I knew at Harvard. After he was contacted by a health-care venture capital group to see if he would be interested in consulting for a new biotechnology company, he approached me and two other Harvard faculty members to see if we would join him on an advisory board. The two others were Dr. Bernard Fields, chairman of microbiology at the Medical School and editor of *Fields Virology*, the bible of viral diseases, and Dr. Mark Greene, an immunologist in the pathology department. The company, called Cambridge Biosciences, was then formed with the four of us on a scientific advisory board. Among the earliest projects were a potential vaccine that veterinarians could use for feline leukemia and diagnostic tests for HTLV and AIDS. The company also negotiated an agreement with Harvard to provide significant funding for research in my laboratory. This filled an important gap for funding our lab activities, as the US government under Reagan was very reluctant to support AIDS research.

In May 1984, about a year after the first bolus of papers were published, Gallo had another set of papers in *Science* that would dramatically advance our knowledge about the cause of AIDS.

chapter ten

Proof of Cause

In May 1984, about a year after the *Science* papers that showed an association with an HTLV-type virus, Gallo's group published four more papers that made a very good case for proof of cause.[66–69] They described the isolation of a new virus they called HTLV-III from 47 cases of either AIDS or pre-AIDS lymphadenopathy-type patients. Antibodies to the new virus were also found in 78–88% of patients with AIDS or pre-AIDS and in 6 of 17 sexual partners of AIDS patients, but in only 1 of 188 controls. By electron microscopy, the virus seemed to resemble the one Montagnier described a year earlier in two patients.[61] Montagnier's group described their virus as LAV, for lymphadenopathy-associated virus. Soon after, most agreed that the viruses were the same, and the designation HTLV-III/LAV was then used. It would take a year or two for most of the scientific and public health communities to digest the information and accept that the cause of AIDS had been established. Other reports in *Science* and elsewhere soon confirmed and extended the data that associated HTLV-III with AIDS. A serological laboratory test was soon devised with whole virus to use for diagnosis of AIDS.

As all of this was going on, we turned some of our attention to hemophiliacs. We had the HTLV-III virus from Gallo and used two different tests to check for antibodies. Of three hemophiliacs with AIDS, all were positive. But of even greater importance, 30 of 47 (64%) asymptomatic hemophiliacs were also positive for the antibodies.[70] None of the controls were positive, but a shocking

94% of hemophiliacs who received unscreened blood before 1984 were positive. It was horrifying to observe results suggesting that most of the hemophiliacs in the United States might have already become infected by the time blood could be screened to prevent the infection. Ultimately, about half of the 10,000 US hemophiliacs would die of AIDS.

In another study with Dr. Joan Kreiss in Los Angeles, we found 2 of 21 (9.5%) wives of HTLV-III antibody–positive hemophiliacs were themselves positive, one of the first leads that heterosexual transmission might also occur.[71] In other studies with Gallo and Dr. Jerry Groopman, we found more cases of apparent heterosexual transmission of HTLV-III. As documented AIDS cases expanded from an epidemic in the United States that was primarily in homosexual men and injection drug users, it would soon be recognized as a world pandemic in which most of the cases in sub-Saharan Africa and Southeast Asia would be associated with heterosexual exposure. As the epidemic spread very rapidly in Africa, it outpaced the epidemics in the United States and Europe. Worldwide, about 90% of the AIDS cases were believed to be heterosexually transmitted by about 1990.

Our lab also spent much time isolating and characterizing the major surface protein of the virus, which we believed to be the piece of the virus that most consistently elicited antibodies. As such, it would presumably be the most important reagent for tests to diagnose AIDS patients and to screen blood to allow safe transfusions and safe production of factor VIIII needed by hemophiliacs. We used the techniques of radiolabel amino acid sequencing and radioimmunoprecipitation to identify viral surface proteins and verify that they fit the appropriate gene sequence for the RNA code of the viral genome.[72,73] The proteins would be named gp120 and gp160, respectively, for the forms found in the virus and in infected cells. The "gp" is for glycoprotein, which is a more elaborate form of the protein that is also linked to a complex carbohydrate. In related studies, we identified other proteins that we could map to specific genes of the HTLV-III genome. We also collected data on how often antibodies were produced to these proteins by infected people. Some seemed good to include in assay systems, but none were as good as the gp120. These studies were done in our lab by Dr. Francis Barin, one of the French virologists that Dr. Philippe Maupas originally sent to our lab to encourage collaboration with his group at the University of Tours.

The gp120 test, which would eventually be identified as the gold standard by the World Health Organization for AIDS diagnosis and blood safety, would also be submitted as a patent application by Harvard officials. Major pharmaceutical companies like Abbott and international agencies like the World Health Organization would recommend the test for use throughout the world. We also adapted the test so it could be used with saliva, which is sometimes more available than blood. A Harvard dental student, David Archibald, conducted this research in my lab as part of his PhD thesis.

Recognition by the medical community that the cause of AIDS had been found and a diagnostic test was about to be available set off a wave of interest by academic institutions and the press. Gallo and I and a few others had more invitations to speak about our research than we could possibly accept. By this time, both of us had large enough research groups of talented people to do much of the lab work, but we still had to talk with the students and fellows almost every day – and this was before the widespread availability of cell phones. I recall one invitation to Argentina to speak at a meeting of a South American medical association. They offered two first-class tickets as an added incentive so I could bring my wife. Elizabeth wasn't interested in going so far for such a brief trip, but Holly, my oldest daughter, was happy to go on the 3-day trip. I gave my talk, we had a couple of good meals, went to the zoo, and flew right back to Boston.

The mid-1980s were the busiest time of my life. Along with conducting the research and teaching, I'd publish 20–25 research papers and take 40 or more trips each year. I never did a medical internship, but I learned to appreciate how it must have felt to work 80 or more hours per week. On one 11-day trip, I went to Houston, then to two cities in South Africa, to Hong Kong and Shanghai, then to Paris, to Los Angeles, back to Paris, and finally back to Boston. I was beyond the concept of jet lag, simply sleeping whenever I could regardless of whether it was day or night. While I was traveling, Elizabeth took care of our daughters and other family members, and worked at her veterinary practice, covering our home front.

On another trip, I traveled from Boston to Honolulu to lecture at a medical meeting on a Friday. I told them I would do it if they could also book my ticket to go through New Zealand on the way back so I could visit Wellington on the weekend. I later realized it was an 8-hour trip from Honolulu to New Zealand. My youngest daughter, Carrie, was there as a high school exchange student. I went there for 1½ days to be with her and to meet her host parents. They thought I was crazy for not staying longer when I had traveled so far, remarking that I was the first person they had met who came to New Zealand for a weekend. I also went to Europe often to speak at scientific meetings. NATO was a frequent sponsor of meetings organized by the Germans. The site they favored was Greece. One time, a Harvard administrator familiar with my travel asked how I liked Greece, noticing that I had been there three times in the last 4 years. He asked about the Parthenon. I realized I had never seen it, except at a great distance, as I had always flown directly from the airport in Athens to the site of the conference, usually Crete or Corfu.

As we gained knowledge, it didn't seem to make things easier for high-risk groups, especially gay men. Many of our university lectures were open to the public, the press, and protesters. On one occasion, I was giving a lecture at the Lyndon B Johnson Memorial Library auditorium at the University of Texas in Austin and was surprised by the response. I presented data from our lab that led us to identify an HTLV-related antibody response and discussed why the first wave of results seemed tantalizing but unclear about establishing cause. I then showed slides about Gallo's results finding HTLV-III and how we identified and then characterized the glycoprotein that would now allow hospital labs to obtain a definitive diagnosis of AIDS or pre-AIDS and test blood to assure that safe transfusions could be made. I concluded with epidemiologic data about the fractions of different populations that were at risk for infection. My host gave some brief comments of praise and thanks, and there was applause. He then asked for questions from the audience. I responded to a few technical questions and noticed that something seemed to be brewing in the back of the hall. The next questioner asked, in a harsh tone, "What are you doing to develop a drug against the AIDS virus?" As he asked the question, a group of 10–15 others got up with signs and placards about how government and university officials were discriminating against homosexuals and causing deaths by their inaction. I could have stated that I agreed with his comments about the government, but I responded that I was not doing drug research because I did not have that expertise. But I was trying to make better diagnostics and better clinical monitoring tests, and I had just started research to explore the possibility of making a vaccine. He responded by shouting, "That's irresponsible, you're a part of the problem, you have some expertise but you're doing nothing to help us!" The host broke in and said, "That's all, this session is over," just as the campus police were pushing their way in. I was shaken and could not understand what I had done to bring this on. Then two other protesters dropped their signs, came up to me, and one quietly said, "Look, we're very sorry for this and apologize to you. We all very much appreciate your research, but you have to understand that the press and local officials pay no attention to us unless we cause a ruckus. Please don't think that any of this is directed to you." They offered to buy me a drink, and I would have taken them up on it except that I had a dinner appointment with my host and his guests. At dinner, I recounted my experience and suggested that university officials set up a dialogue with the protesters.

In another instance, I went to New York City to give a lecture at the Memorial Sloan Kettering Cancer Center. It was before we had newspapers online, and there were many newsstands at busy pedestrian crossings in the city. As I went around the corner to enter the building, I noticed a tabloid with a full front-page headline that read, "Should Gallo and Essex Be in Jail? AIDSGate Begins." It was in a bimonthly paper called the *New York Native*. I hadn't heard of it before. It apparently was put out by gay activists in New York, and the title was in reference to an editorial by the editor, Charles Ortleb. His issue was that Gallo had not collaborated sufficiently with Luc Montagnier in France. The allegation against me was that I had been a longtime collaborator with Gallo and "remained silent" about the need for Gallo to collaborate with Montagnier. Ortleb was described as a crackpot, and the paper was known for their stories on denial that HIV was the cause of AIDS and for various conspiracy theories. The paper was denounced and boycotted by some other gay activists in New York, such as ACT UP, a group that ultimately had a positive effect by forcing political leaders to support more research. Nevertheless, as I was introduced for the talk at Sloan Kettering, the man introducing me mentioned that he had just seen my name in the newspaper headlines. Acknowledging why was certainly not the easiest way to begin a lecture.

Funding for AIDS research had still not caught up with the need to expand our knowledge on AIDS and explore both the many needs of US patients and the burgeoning worldwide pandemic. Even though Reagan had still not mentioned AIDS by the end of his first term, the National Institutes of Health started to fund research grants. The National Cancer Institute became interested because many AIDS patients developed Kaposi sarcoma and opportunistic lymphomas. The National Institute of Heart, Lung, and Blood became interested in protecting the blood supply and because of the opportunistic pneumonias. And the National Institute of Allergy and Infectious Diseases became interested because they had jurisdiction for both opportunistic infectious diseases and for immunology in general. Dr. Tony Fauci, their new director, took great interest in the research.

By chance, the National Cancer Institute started a new program in 1985 for funding research grant proposals. The usual process was that each applicant had to submit a project proposal with a hypothesis, specific aims, and detailed methods. Funding was usually for up to $150,000 per year for 3 years, occasionally for 5 years. At the time, I had three ongoing grants of this type. The new program, called "Outstanding Investigator Grants," could award up to $1,000,000 per year for 7 years to a small number of applicants. It was designed for proven scientists who already had a record of original discoveries. Not only was it for more money, the application process was much simpler as well. The applicant only had to project the general directions and plans, without specifying details or methods. The reviewers decided that I was "one of the leading scientists in the biomedical community," which was all I needed to get the grant. To top it off, I was also allowed to be a part of other applications if the application agency decided I was necessary for the program. The National Heart, Lung, and Blood Institute had a new mechanism for medical institutions to apply for program research support on blood safety to cover HTLV, hepatitis B, and HTLV-III/LAV. In pre-application discussions, the NIH and Harvard personnel decided that participation by both me and one of my associates, Dr. Tun-Hou Lee, might be necessary for the success of the program, even though I already had the NCI Outstanding Investigator Grant. We agreed to participate, and it gave us more research funding. The timing was important. At the earliest stage, our lab was probably the only one at Harvard with experience studying HTLV and HTLV-III. If it had been a year or two later, there might have been several more who were qualified.

In 1986, the Lasker Award, the highest award for medical research in the United States, was awarded to Bob Gallo, Luc Montagnier, and me. It is sometimes thought of as the "American Nobel." The Lasker Foundation seems to take pride in identifying and celebrating the next generation of scientific discoveries. About half of the Lasker Award recipients go on to receive the Nobel Prize. Montagnier did, in 2008. In my humble opinion, Gallo deserved it more than Montagnier, and more than me, for that matter. The Lasker Award was for discoveries that helped determine the cause of AIDS. In Gallo's case and Montagnier's, the award was for the discovery of the virus. In my case, it was for showing that retroviruses could cause immunosuppression, in the case of cats, and for developing the gp120 test to diagnose AIDS.

The Lasker Awards are presented at a luncheon in New York City with up to 300 people in attendance. Many are representatives of major organizations interested in medical research, including foundations and pharmaceutical companies. An added benefit in receiving the award is the introduction to the Lasker board members, who in many cases help identify resources for the recipients. Soon after returning home, I had a phone call from Mrs. Mary

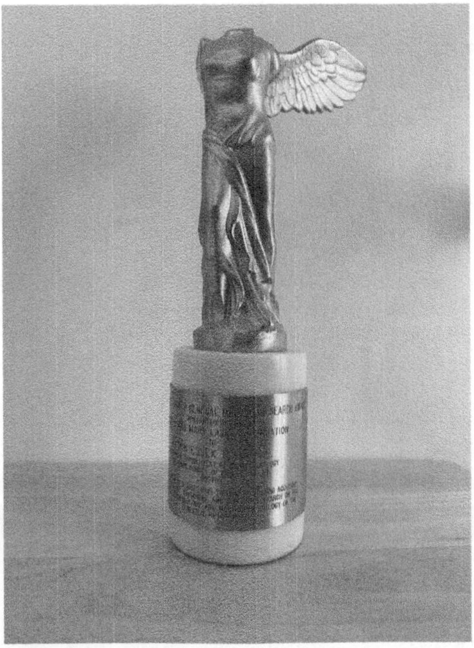

Figure 10.1: Lasker Award

Lasker and Mrs. Deeda Blair, a vice president of the foundation, to say that I would be receiving a grant to support my plan to begin research on AIDS in Africa.

In 1986, a subcommittee of the International Committee on Taxonomy of Viruses recommended a change to the name of the AIDS virus, from HTLV-III and/or LAV to HIV, for human immunodeficiency virus. Both Bob Gallo and I were on the committee, and we both voted against the name change. Gallo voted against it because he had introduced the HTLV-III term to follow the names for HTLV-I and HTLV-II, both of which he had initially identified. In the HTLV-I term, the "L" was to be for leukemia, which that virus caused, but he argued that the "L" could equally well refer to "lymphotropic," as all the viruses infected and did their pathology to T lymphocytes. Both Gallo and I had already published more than a few papers using the term HTLV-III and

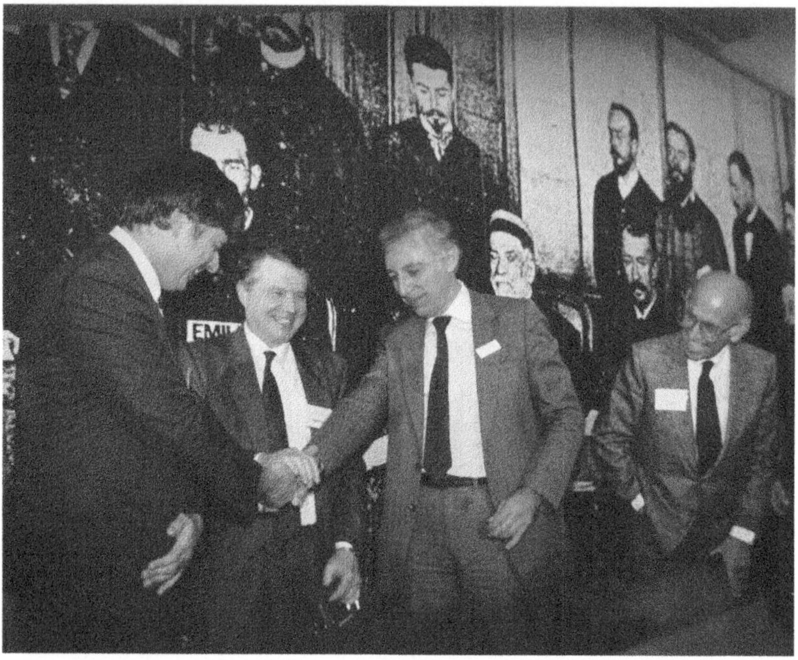

Figure 10.2: Max Essex, Luc Montagnier, Bob Gallo, Jonas Salk

felt that introducing a new term now would cause more confusion than benefit. The majority of the people on the committee did not work with the human retroviruses. I was also opposed to the name change for an even more complex reason. Dr. Phyllis Kanki in our group had just discovered two new viruses related to HTLV-III. One, which we found in people in West Africa, had already been referred to in very recent publications as HTLV-IV.[74] The second, which we found in monkeys, we had initially called the simian T cell lymphotropic virus, STLV or STLV-III, because it was cross-reactive with HTLV-III in serologic tests and clearly related to it.[75] In retrospect, although confusing for a 2–3 year period, coalescing around the term HIV was probably less confusing in the long term. The new virus we called HTLV-IV would subsequently be named HIV-2.

chapter eleven

AIDS in Africa

In July 1981, my wife Elizabeth and I were in Taipei, Taiwan, where I had been invited to speak at the National Medical Association annual meeting. The first day of the meeting had speeches by myself and two other international guests who were also invited with their wives. After the first day of talks, we and the other international guests were invited to spend 2–3 days at Sun Moon Lake, a resort area about 2 hours away. One of the other guests was Dr. Christiaan Barnard, the famous heart surgeon from South Africa who did the first heart transplant in the world in 1967. In the 1970s medical community, Barnard seemed to have an almost rock star type of image. While we were secluded at the resort, the royal wedding of Diana, Princess of Wales, and then Prince Charles was on TV. Dr. Barnard pulled me aside for a long walk during which he confided about the pressure he was under because of the visibility of his work. The next day he invited me to go to the University of Cape Town as his guest. I decided to go as I had never been to South Africa. In 1982, I traveled to Cape Town via an airline called Union Transport D. The plane was mainly for cargo, but it had a small number of passenger seats. The apartheid government of South Africa was cut off from most countries in Africa, except for Congo, where we stopped for fuel. After arrival in Cape Town, I received VIP status as a guest of Dr. Barnard and was impressed by his vast wards of experimental pigs with transplanted hearts. However, the government-directed racial separation, which would go on until the early 1990s, was shocking. An old protester friend from my California days, Dr. Fritz van der Riet, took me to visit the Black slums at Crossroads. It was depressing. Years later, I'd get to have lunch with President Mandela and appreciate firsthand why he became such a beloved and great leader. Unfortunately, that also happened at a time when the Republic of South Africa would lead the world as the country with the most AIDS cases.

By 1983, there were quite a few reports of people coming to Europe when they were already infected with HIV. The most frequent reports were for people coming from francophone countries in Africa. One report referred to a man from Central Africa infecting a dozen or more individuals in Belgium. By 1985, it was clear that quite a few people were already infected in countries such as Zaire, Côte d'Ivoire, and Uganda. Unlike the situation in the United States and Europe, where homosexual contact among men was important, it seemed that the vast majority of transmissions in Africa were from heterosexual contact, and women had rates of infection that were as high as men's, perhaps even higher. Injection drug use also seemed unimportant in Africa. Blood transfusion may have had a small role in some places where the practice was common for people who had anemia from malaria.

The situation in Africa raised some obvious questions. Why was the epidemic there overwhelmingly one of heterosexual transmission when the AIDS epidemic in Europe and the United States was mainly in homosexual men? Or, alternatively, why hadn't there been more of a heterosexual epidemic in the United States and Europe or more homosexual infections in men in Africa? Could the lack of a male homosexual epidemic in Africa be just because male homosexuals are even more hidden there because of political and governmental oppression? The latter might be important, especially in countries that had barbaric laws about homosexuality, like Uganda. But several studies were done later with male homosexuals in Africa, and their rates of infection were usually at or below the levels seen in heterosexuals in the same countries. Another question was why more cases of HIV infection were not found in general hospital or clinic patients, as hypodermic needles and syringes were often used without complete sterilization and disposable syringes were not as readily available as in the United

States. This could perhaps be because needles in poor African settings were usually thoroughly flushed with water before reuse. With injection drug use, the syringes and needles are often passed directly between participants, resulting in "mini-transfusions." Questions also came up about whether mosquitoes might transmit HIV. This was soon dismissed, in part because there was no correlation between AIDS and mosquito bites in areas where mosquito-borne malaria is common.

My hypothesis for the sexual differences in HIV infection rates included the possibility of HIV strain or subtype differences. We and others would later find some partial evidence for this.[76] Behavioral changes associated with postcolonial mobility and demographics, as well as other sexually transmitted infections, may also have played a role in the very rapid expansion of the HIV epidemic in sub-Saharan Africa. Young adults often move to cities with expanding urbanization. Buses and automobiles, along with road-building, allow for more rapid dissemination of pathogens. Industrialization and air travel may also have been important. It is possible to imagine that a zoonotic virus newly entering the human population might have a tougher time expanding beyond the first cohort if it entered in an isolated village, just as people in the isolated villages might have closer proximity to infected animals than those in urban areas. The most mobile populations and occupations, like young adults who were truck drivers or soldiers, often had the highest rates of HIV infection, as did female sex workers. Fortunately, perhaps, at about the same time world populations became more mobile, we also had a massive expansion in medical knowledge. This was particularly true for the new tools of molecular biology and genetics that allow us to understand new infectious diseases and what to do about them much more rapidly.

As more women became infected and more pregnant women revealed the infection, maternal transmission to infants emerged as another horrendous problem. Although we would later develop effective procedures to prevent almost all maternal transmissions, through both *in utero*[77] and postnatal[78] mechanisms, these measures would only become available years later, after millions of children had already become infected. Delivery by Cesarean section done in a sterilized environment as in the United States or Europe for reduction of HIV transmission was generally not available in Africa. Untreated sexually transmitted diseases like syphilis or gonorrhea also appear to facilitate transmission of HIV, whether by heterosexual or mother–infant contact. A lack of circumcision of men is also modestly associated with sexual transmission. The use of condoms, when available, reduces transmission.

The development of lab tests for HIV, especially simple commercially available tests, made tracking the epidemic in Africa easier to achieve, at least if governmental officials allowed such studies to be done. In the early stages, several African leaders were in denial about the presence of AIDS in their country or region. Some, like some officials in the West, were motivated by fear. Other African leaders were concerned about economic issues, both industrial development and safari tourism. At the same time, leaders in some other countries like Botswana, Namibia, and Senegal were very open about AIDS, even seeking collaboration and advice from outsiders, including myself and others.

In late 1985, the World Health Organization (WHO) brought together a small group of AIDS researchers and physicians, myself included, and charged us with developing a new and better definition for African AIDS. Earlier clinical definitions for AIDS, developed by such groups as the US Centers for Disease Control and Prevention and the US military, were based on the signs and symptoms seen in Western patients. Although the most fundamental feature of AIDS in any population is immune suppression, particularly a loss of T cells, clinical or hospital laboratory testing to make this diagnosis was not available in most clinics in Africa. Testing for the presence of HIV was becoming more available, and a profile of signs and symptoms and sick people with HIV could be developed.

I flew from Brussels to Kinshasa, Zaire, where I stayed for 2 days, then crossed the Congo River in a rickety ferry and went by auto to Bangui in the Central African Republic. While in Kinshasa, I visited some AIDS wards at the Mama Yemo Hospital. One ward had more than a dozen emaciated women on makeshift cots, all with advanced brain infections and near death. The people in Kinshasa and Bangui seemed astonishingly poor. In Kinshasa, I also met with two physician-pathologists. One, Dr. Oscar Kashala, seemed to be remarkably bright and ambitious but also a kind and caring person. He had just received notice about getting a 5-year financial grant from the WHO to study infectious diseases and oncology anywhere in Europe or the United States. Based on his international test scores, he was accepted for a PhD program at Harvard while doing his research in my lab. Years later, he would run for president of the Democratic Republic of Congo, formerly known as Zaire. Oscar's mentor in Kinshasa, Dr. Raphael Kalengayi, also impressed me as a warm and devoted teacher who had learned all he could about the local AIDS epidemic. I was so impressed with him that I invited him, along with our friend in Senegal, Dr. Souleymane Mboup, and my collaborators in Boston, Drs. Phyllis Kanki and Ric Marlink, to join me as co-editors of a book series on AIDS in Africa.[79]

When arriving in Kinshasa, I made the mistake of converting some of my US dollars to the local currency called "zaires." The inflation had been so steep that I could barely fit all the paper currency I got for $60 into my pockets. I then splurged for a dinner of crocodile steak with two friends.

It was unclear why the WHO selected the Central African Republic as the site to develop a definition for African AIDS. The country is between Sudan and Congo, mainly within the Ubangi River basin. It has very few tourists, perhaps a few to visit the Bayaka pygmy peoples, and has been listed as the unhealthiest country in the world. Currently in a 12-year civil war, it has had a series of dictators, perhaps the most brutal being Bokassa, the self-proclaimed emperor also known as the "butcher of Bangui." Fortunately, he was ousted by the French a few years before our visit. A brief visit to the local outdoor market gave me an appreciation for the lack of adequate nutrition. It had about 15–20 tables of items for sale. A few were "bush meat" of unknown origin, potatoes, or yams. More than half the tables sold only dried caterpillars or grubs. I tried to take a photo of one table, but the salesperson jumped in front and indicated I could not. I then offered her a coin, and she nodded yes while I took the photo of her next to the table. She then swept about 15 piles of the grubs into a large paper sack and handed it to me. I took it back to my hotel. The grubs didn't seem very appetizing, so I left the sack in my room as a tip. On our last night in Bangui, our WHO leader indicated that he had arranged a dinner at the home of a local woman who was renowned for her cooking skills. Following the local cuisine, we had barbecued meat with yams and maize. We all ate our fill and then learned it was monkey meat, but it had been well cooked.

The WHO/Bangui clinical definition for African AIDS was developed not just because lab tests for T cell counts were not often available but also because some of the opportunistic infections that were most common in the West, like Pneumocystis, are not commonly found in the African environment. Others, like cryptococcosis, are more common in Africa, resulting in a higher fraction of meningitis in AIDS cases. Tuberculosis is more prevalent in Africa, especially the species of Mycobacterium that is most common in people with pulmonary disease. In the United States, Mycobacterium avis, the species that is found primarily in birds, is the most common cause of pulmonary tuberculosis in AIDS patients but extremely rare in patients who do not have HIV-type immunosuppression. Another presentation that seems more common for AIDS in Africa is "wasting" or severe weight loss. Some early presentations like lymphadenopathy and oral thrush are seen in both US and African patients. Overall, however, a major advancement in the African AIDS definition is the inclusion of an HIV-positive test. While beneficial for clinical diagnosis and epidemic monitoring, the denialists try to use the HIV-positive test as a negative criterion, arguing that the HIV infection itself is therefore not causal. This is why the lab demonstration of T cell immunosuppression is the most important indicator of the fundamental disease state, just as the inability to make or regulate insulin is the basis for the disease we call diabetes.

Both in Africa and in the West, infection with HIV is often followed by an acute phase of a mononucleosis-like illness within 2–5 weeks. This is characterized by a rapid expansion of HIV replication with high levels of virus in the blood, called viremia. The patients are highly infectious to others at this stage, but in almost all cases, the symptoms are temporarily resolved and the viremia greatly reduced. Some patients show no symptoms, but all seem to have some level of viremia. Most patients then show no disease symptoms for 3–6 years, then gradually deteriorate, beginning with lymphadenopathy and ending with the lethal infectious diseases. If the populations at risk are highly mobile, it is easy to see how infected individuals could spread the infections before displaying AIDS symptoms. When patients develop late-stage symptoms, they again have high levels of viremia and transmissibility. But at that stage, they are much less likely to be sexually active or to donate blood, so they present less risk for infecting others.

Different regions of Africa have had different levels of impact from the epidemic of HIV/AIDS. Some differences may be based on social practices or governmental policies, but there are also differences based on viral subtypes and geographical region. North Africa, like most of the Middle East, has not had a major impact from HIV. Central and East Africa appeared to have the most severe impact by the late 1980s, with high or very high rates in places like Uganda, Zaire, Rwanda, Burundi, and the Republic of Congo with well-documented epidemics. By the late 1980s, most countries in southern Africa had not experienced a severe epidemic, except, perhaps, for countries like Zambia or Tanzania that border Central Africa. But a decade or more later, southern African countries would have the highest rates of HIV infection in the world. As for West Africa, most countries had relatively low rates except for Côte d'Ivoire, which had higher rates.

In the mid- to late 1980s, azidothymidine (AZT), also called zidovudine (ZVD), first became available in the West. It was not generally available in Africa, but it usually only prolongs the life of AIDS patients for 6–8 months. The very effective combinations of drugs that saved lives started to become available in the West by the mid- to late 1990s. They would not become available in most of Africa until much later. In 2002, Dr. Jeff Sachs, then a Harvard economics professor, organized a letter campaign with several other Harvard faculty, including myself, to demand that the more effective drugs be made available in Africa. The President's Emergency Plan for AIDS Relief (PEPFAR), which President George W. Bush began in 2003, would eventually have a major impact, saving at least 25 million lives, primarily by offering drug treatment.

In many places in Africa, there were programs to prevent infections. Some programs to reduce partners and use condoms were partially effective. But many African women want to have children, even at a young age, so condom use was difficult to promote in those populations. In the KwaZulu-Natal region of South Africa, teenage girls got infected at very high rates. Some behavioral projects even offered girls a stipend to stay in school as a deterrent to sexual promiscuity. In Africa, as in so many other places, stigma and discrimination were also major problems for those who became infected.

HIV/AIDS also had a major impact on economic development in Africa. It was more than just a health problem. Health-care personnel were sometimes diverted from routine maternal care and administration of infant vaccines to care for dying AIDS patients. HIV caused a depletion of teachers, police, and military personnel in some countries. Infection rates were more associated with mobility than with poverty. In some countries, the most educated had higher rates of HIV infection.

By the mid-1980s, our research group decided we must get involved in Africa. We began in Senegal.

chapter twelve

Senegal and HIV-2

Senegal is an interesting country with charming people. It sits on the westernmost edge of the African continent. The land shelf drops off to deep water very rapidly from Dakar, the largest city, so fishermen sometimes catch very big fish within sight of the shoreline. Wolof is the language spoken most often, but all the educated people also speak French. A subset of the people are very tall, including Abdou Diouf at 6′6′, who was president from 1985 to 2000, and Tacko Fall at 7′5′, who played for the Boston Celtics basketball team. After my first introduction to Senegal by Dr. Philippe Maupas to participate in a hepatitis workshop, I was reintroduced by Dr. Jean-Loup Romet-Lemonne, a former Maupas trainee who subsequently joined our research group in Boston.

Jean-Loup suggested we partner with Dr. Souleymane Mboup, an up-and-coming energetic faculty member at Cheikh Anta Diop University Medical School in Dakar. After we established the partnership in 1985, I and several others in the Harvard team became close friends with Souleymane for the next 30–40 years, together publishing hundreds of scientific articles. He spoke no English when we first met. Within a year, he was fluent in English.

Our mutual plan was to collect blood samples from as many people as possible and to screen them for antibodies to HIV. We soon realized that Dakar had a large population of female sex workers, a population that usually has the highest rates of infections with viruses and other microbes that might be sexually transmitted. We also discovered that most of the sex workers had permits to practice sex work in exchange for compliance with governmental guidelines. To remain legal, the prostitutes had to agree to semiannual health exams. Souleymane soon succeeded in getting the Senegalese government to add an HIV antibody test to the 6-month exam. Our research group would take responsibility for the HIV test and the health exams, and invite the women to enroll in a research cohort to evaluate incidence or rates of new infections, as well as health outcomes. Working with Souleymane and Dr. Phyllis Kanki of our lab group, Dr. Ibou Thior was put in charge of the sex worker cohort. Ibou, a physician by training, would later go on to earn a graduate degree in epidemiology at Harvard and become the first on-site head of the Harvard program in Botswana. The sex worker cohort in Senegal would remain in place for about two decades.

Many of the female sex workers were not native to Dakar or even Senegal, as a significant proportion had migrated through other francophone countries in West Africa. Some were from as far away as Côte d'Ivoire. We soon learned that women from the southern or Casamance region of Senegal had the highest rates of HIV infection. But oddly, the virus that infected these women seemed different, only partially cross-reactive with HIV by antibody tests. And almost all of the infected women seemed healthy, not showing any clinical signs of AIDS or even preclinical lymphadenopathy. We decided we had to learn more about the population there, so we took the once-per-week flight on Air Senegal to Ziguinchor, the only major town in the area, which was right on the border of Guinea-Bissau. We succeeded in collecting quite a few samples in the area and learned that most of the sex workers moved around between the Casamance region of southern Senegal and the northern region of Guinea-Bissau, even going back to Bissau, the capital city, on a regular basis.

After a few days in Ziguinchor, we were ready to go back to Dakar so we could process and test the blood samples. Assuming we'd have to wait 2 days for a scheduled flight, we were happy to learn that a chartered plane would be there in the afternoon and that they had three open seats to accommodate us. Upon boarding, we learned that the flight had been chartered to pick up survivors of a large tanker shipwreck that had gone down off the north coast of Guinea-Bissau a few days before. We learned that the group of 15 included 12 Portuguese crew workers and a first mate from Lisbon, a Greek captain, and a New York insurance agent who had just flown in to meet the crew. The freighter had been carrying sugarcane along the African coast and selectively moving between countries that were former Portuguese colonies – Mozambique, Angola, Guinea-Bissau, and Cape Verde. Later, it would help us understand why a particular virus seemed to be present at significant levels in these countries but not in most others.

We were surprised by what we found in the Senegalese blood samples. The antibodies from the sex workers reacted with the HIV virus, but they reacted even better with an HIV-related monkey virus we called the simian immunodeficiency virus, or SIV. It almost seemed as if the people were infected with the monkey virus rather than HIV. In earlier studies, we had found a virus related to the human leukemia virus HTLV in Asian macaque monkeys with leukemia or lymphoma.[42] Soon after, we found a second virus in macaques with AIDS-like illnesses. We called this one SIV because it was more closely related to HIV than to HTLV.[80] As we found new information in both monkeys and people, it seemed to expand the number of questions we had to answer. Why was a virus that was in research colonies of at least some species of Asian monkeys also in human populations in West Africa?

We decided we had to catch and test some African monkeys. Monkeys seem to be a very successful species in Africa, especially the African green monkey, or vervet. They are medium-sized and found all over sub-Saharan Africa in colonies of 20 or more. They have learned to be aggressive scavengers of human food. I recall one instance where a vervet grabbed an apple from the hand of a picnicking child. I also remember a time when Elizabeth and I were having an outside lunch at the home of some friends, Michelle and Chris Schaan, in Gaborone, Botswana. Monkeys were throwing mangoes at us from a tree above the table and squawking loudly. Michelle assumed they were upset because her dog RK (his full name was Road Kill because Chris had rescued him on the street following an auto accident) was at the end of the table. Michelle put RK in the house, and the monkeys were then quiet.

As soon as we spoke at scientific meetings about the SIV virus that infected colonized Asian macaques with an AIDS-like illness, some colleagues who had research colonies of African green monkeys contacted us and offered us samples to check. We found that up to two-thirds of the research colony green monkeys had apparent infections with SIV but no AIDS-like disease.[81] But we still had to determine if the viruses were in wild African monkeys in West Africa, where the sex workers were infected with the SIV-related HIV.

Souleymane then recruited monkey hunters. Monkeys are a common form of "bush meat" consumed by some Africans. They are not shot but rather caught in traps and maintained alive until butchering and consumption because of the lack of refrigeration. To catch the monkeys, the hunter digs a deep hole in the earth with an adjacent top screen that would be propped up and tied to a line that the hunter holds while hiding behind a bush. Some fruit or grain is left around the hole with even more at the bottom of the hole. After one or more monkeys jump into the hole, the hunter drops the screen to trap them. Getting the animals out is the biggest challenge, and the hunters are often bitten. This has sometimes been cited as a possible "spillover" step where the zoonotic monkey SIV can get transmitted to the human population. It seems to me that an even more likely "spillover" interspecies transmission might happen when the butcher, hands covered with viremic monkey blood, might accidentally cut himself with a sharp knife. Either way, it seems that such interspecies transmissions might have happened multiple times, as the human SIV-related virus in one geographical setting often seems genetically closer to the local monkey virus than either does to the human and monkey viruses found a few hundred miles away. Yet the human and monkey viruses at the site a few hundred miles away would also be close to each other.

We also wondered how the Asian monkeys and research colonies got infected, especially when we found that various samples we checked from wild Asian macaques in different locations were virus free. The only hypothesis that seemed to make sense was that the colonized research monkeys were either exposed to infected African monkeys in the research facility or exposed to blood or other tissues from West African people at a Western/US research facility. It was known that some of the research colony Asian monkeys were injected with blood from human malaria patients, and such human blood, especially from West Africans, could have harbored the monkey-like HIV as well. Senegal, in fact, is a site where malaria is endemic, as are many other places in Africa. If it were human materials injected into the Asian lab monkeys that caused the first outbreak of an AIDS-like disease in these monkeys, it would be an example of a reverse "spillover."[82] This would be the opposite of the direct spillover often used as the explanation for how SARS-CoV-2 moved from animals in the "wet markets" of Wuhan, China, to start the current worldwide pandemic.[83]

We would also need an explanation for why the "same" monkey virus might cause an AIDS-like disease in Asian monkeys but no obvious disease in African green monkeys. However, this could be explained, at least as a hypothesis, through evolutionary "survival of the fittest," whereas the Asian monkeys would have been first introduced to the virus only one or a few generations ago. An analogous situation might be the monkey herpesviruses, saimiri and ateles, as mentioned in chapter 2. In the monkey species where those viruses are endemic in nature, the viruses appear to exist as a harmless commensal infection, whereas in another monkey species, they cause a rapidly lethal lymphoma. It is well known that one can select "strains" of laboratory mice for near lethality or disease from some viruses by selecting the least fit as breeding parents for the next generation. In mice, this might only take a few years because of their rapid generation time. For monkeys, it would obviously take longer.

While the monkey studies were intellectually interesting, we realized that we must do much more to study the new SIV-like virus in the people of West Africa. We hired a young French physician, Dr. Dominique Ricard, to move around Senegal to collect more human blood samples. Dominique, like many of our younger recruits from the Maupas group in Tours, France, had served a year or two in the French army, stationed in former French colonies like the Central African Republic, Côte d'Ivoire, and Senegal. Those with such a background seemed to function very well as members of our research team. We dispatched Dominique to go to all major cities in Senegal but to concentrate on collecting the most human blood samples from the Casamance region in the south, as that is where we had found the origin of many of the sex workers and also where the people had the highest prevalence of the new SIV-like human virus.

Dominique usually traveled by motor scooter, even between rural villages where the most direct route might be little more than a dirt path between the dense growth of bush. On one occasion, he got into an accident as he ran into a python, a large snake lying across the dirt path. It was so long that he could not get around the snake. He braked, but not soon enough, and he flew over the bike and the snake when he hit it, damaging his shoulder. Fortunately, the snake just ambled away, but when we submitted the accident report to cover Dominique's hospital expenses, the Harvard insurance office questioned the accuracy of the report. It could have been much worse, as the rock python is one of the largest snakes in the world and known to be aggressive. On another occasion when I was driving a small truck on a dirt road, another snake was lying across the road. I waited 5–10 minutes, and when it didn't move, I tried nudging it with the truck. It responded by attacking the truck tire that had nudged it. We then rolled up all the windows and waited for it to leave on its own. Such snakes have now become a source of bush meat in many countries, sometimes a delicacy. I remember a restaurant in southern Senegal that had a large dead python draped over the sign at the doorway, presumably to entice diners.

We found the SIV-related HIV in many more people. About 40% of the sex workers in Ziguinchor were infected, but only 0.4% were infected with HIV-1. Those infected with the monkey-related virus were rarely ill. Eventually, the identification of the virus would be confirmed by other research groups from France and Sweden, and also by the US CDC, which had a lab in Abidjan, Côte d'Ivoire. The new virus was then named HIV-2. In Senegal and Guinea-Bissau,

HIV-2 was much more common than HIV-1, but in Abidjan, HIV-1 was more common. Older women had the highest rates of infection with the new virus, which shared about 40–50% of its gene sequence with HIV-1, but the other half of the genome was different. And the genetic diversity within different HIV-2s was less than for HIV-1s.

Later, we determined that HIV-2 spread less efficiently than HIV-1.[84] This was true for both sexual transmission between adults and for vertical transmission from mother to baby. Only 1–2% of babies of HIV-2-infected mothers were themselves infected, but 25–35% of babies born to HIV-1-infected mothers were infected. Over a 15-year period of studying the Dakar sex worker cohort, incidence or rate of new infections stayed about the same. But for HIV-1 incidence, it went up over time. Although discovered later than HIV-1, the HIV-2 was more stable in the population. Evolutionarily, it appeared to be an older virus in the human population, already having reached endemic status.

There also appeared to be a major difference for lethality between HIV-1 and HIV-2.[85] By comparing time of infection in the sex worker cohort, one-third of HIV-1-infected women had clinical AIDS within 5 years after infection, but none of an equal number of HIV-2-infected women had AIDS in 5 years. Looking at blood samples, we found a good explanation. On average, the HIV-1-infected women had 30 times more virus in their body than the HIV-2-infected women had. This was also associated with a more rapid fall in T4 blood lymphocytes in the HIV-1-infected women. As time went on with the cohort of Senegalese sex workers, we also found that a few developed an AIDS-like disease but only after a much longer period of time. Since we could only follow the population for 10–15 years, it was impossible to know whether all the HIV-2-infected people would develop disease if followed for 30–50 years, as almost all of the HIV-1-infected people did within 8–10 years, or if many HIV-2-infected people would remain disease free for a normal lifespan. Studies by others reported rare HIV-2-infected patients in the Boston area and elsewhere. Most of the New England patients came from a population of Cape Verdeans who had settled in the area near Providence, Rhode Island,

and New Bedford, Massachusetts. Other HIV-2 infections were reported in people from Brazil and Goa, a state in western India populated by Portuguese-speaking people, as well as from Portugal itself.

With the recognition that HIV-2 was less likely to cause AIDS and HIV-1 steadily increasing in the Senegalese sex workers, we saw an opportunity to ask another question. Did HIV-2 offer any protection against subsequent infection with HIV-1? Karin Travers, a doctoral student with Phyllis Kanki, found the answer. HIV-2-infected women were less likely to become infected with HIV-1 than were uninfected women.[86] Conversely, if a woman was first infected with HIV-1, this offered no protection against subsequent infection with HIV-2. This in turn stimulated us to try to learn more about this phenomenon; in particular, could the HIV-2-associated protection give us clues about how to make a vaccine for AIDS?

As we began to appreciate the extent of the AIDS problem and the presence of different viruses, one man led a new movement of denialism, claiming that AIDS was not a real disease and that it was not caused by HIV.

chapter thirteen

Duesberg and the Denialists

The saga of Dr. Peter Duesberg might be best characterized as a tragedy. It was a personal tragedy for Duesberg, who left his early career as a cancer researcher to become an AIDS denialist. Though he had never done research on HIV and/or AIDS, in the mid-1980s, he redirected most of his time away from his own research to become a full-time critic of those who were doing AIDS research. His own research plummeted, and he lost grant funding and the academic and scientific respect he had previously enjoyed. Colleagues initially thought of him as unserious, but soon after, as destructive and dangerous. By his own admission, former friends and collaborators avoided him. But he seemed to enjoy the attention as undisputed leader of the denialists. None of his followers were folks who had done any serious experimental research on HIV or AIDS, but they too enjoyed the spotlight occasionally offered by journalists looking for something different. In the big picture, however, Duesberg's 25-year career as an AIDS denialist was a much greater tragedy for patients throughout the world. His teachings played an important role in the deaths of hundreds of thousands of people who were either exposed to or infected with HIV.

There is general agreement that Peter Duesberg was very intelligent. After obtaining his PhD in chemistry in Germany, he went to the University of California at Berkeley as a postdoctoral research fellow. The Department of Molecular Biology there was then one of the top in the world, best known for using bacterial viruses to understand how genes replicate. Along with another junior fellow in the department, Duesberg first discovered a cancer gene, designated "sarc," in a chicken virus.

I first met Peter in the mid-1970s when we were both invited speakers at some of the cancer meetings, especially those focused on retroviruses that might cause cancer. He became intrigued with our research on feline leukemia and invited me to give a talk at Berkeley. He had also been invited to give major lectures at Harvard and MIT. He was known for his quick wit. I recall one time, after I gave a lecture at Berkeley, when he invited me to his home. He lived in a contemporary house on a hillside that overlooked San Francisco Bay. As we walked up to the house, I saw quite a few snails in the grass. Peter said, "I must get Baluda up here to eat them." Marcel Baluda was a mutual friend from France who was then a highly respected retrovirologist at UCLA. Later, as we were sitting on the deck overlooking the bay, Peter said, "Sometimes I like to sit here to watch the boats delivering salt to Bishop and Varmus." Mike Bishop and Harold Varmus were also mutual friends and fellow retrovirologists at the University of California at San Francisco who won the Nobel Prize in 1989 for identifying the cellular oncogene counterpart to Duesberg's chicken virus "sarc" gene. To stretch the sensitivity of the DNA experiments requires high concentrations of salt, but not boatloads.

Long before HIV or AIDS, Duesberg had a reputation as an iconoclast. He was also an excellent debater whose criticism could be destructive to more timid colleagues. In the late 1970s and early 1980s, he and I both served as reviewers for the American Cancer Society. Every 3–4 months, we would meet in New York City with 10–12 other colleagues to review and rank cancer research grant applications to determine who would get funded. Ordinarily, there would be 50 or 60 applications for every 8–10 that could be funded. Each committee member would present 4 or 5 applications to the entire group as the "primary" reviewer. Peter would sometimes begin his commentary by laughing about the applicant's research proposal. The chair of the committee would criticize Duesberg because of his lack of respect for the process and instruct the rest of us to ignore his comments.

In mid-1984, about 3 years after the first description of AIDS, Gallo's set of four papers in *Science* resulted in a general consensus among researchers, physicians, and public health officials that AIDS was a new and distinct disease, and that it was caused by HIV. There was still some confusion about the definition of the disease because of the different types of cancers and infections that might be the final outcome. There was also confusion about the names for HIV, until there was agreement that LAV and HTLV-III were the same virus and that it should be called HIV. There was also consensus that the real disease caused by HIV was immunosuppression, whereby the T4 lymphocytes, sometimes called the director cells of the immune system, were destroyed. The outcomes of TB, pneumonia, and meningitis were just some of the sequelae. It was also confusing to some because the disease happened as a gradual progression over 1–10 years. For the first 5–10 years of his denial, Duesberg refused to accept that there even was such a disease as AIDS. Later, when faced with the situation in Africa, he seemed to accept that such a disease might exist but that it was caused by recreational drugs and/or therapeutic drugs used to treat the HIV infection. He also insisted that HIV, by then shown to be present in essentially all AIDS patients, was a harmless passenger virus that caused no disease. No serious virologists or infectious disease physicians paid much attention to his exhortations, but he did entice dozens of fringe players who became believers in his story.

A sad but illustrative example is the case of Christine Maggiore. Christine was diagnosed with HIV at a health exam in 1992. A former boyfriend also tested positive. She initially became active in AIDS charities and AIDS education in Los Angeles, where she lived. This was at about the same time that drugs against HIV were becoming available and some high-profile patients, like Magic Johnson, were effectively treated. In 1994, Christine met Peter Duesberg and decided that her HIV infection was irrelevant and not related to AIDS. She founded an organization, Alive and Well AIDS Alternatives, whose key message was to deny that HIV caused AIDS. She refused to take antiretroviral drugs that could have saved both her and her daughter, who was breastfed during her positive stage. Both she and her 3-year-old daughter later died with signs and symptoms of AIDS.[87] It is possible that both she and her daughter would be alive if she had never met Duesberg.

To my knowledge, Duesberg has never been a student of pathology or epidemiology. These disciplines bring a complexity to infectious diseases that may be difficult to comprehend if one's training is limited to chemistry or mathematics. The definition of the word "cause" becomes more functional, less esoteric. All epidemiologists I know strongly believe that lung cancer is caused by cigarette smoking, and not only because one of their own, Sir Richard Doll, was a pioneer in demonstrating this relationship. But no epidemiologist would state that all cigarette smokers, even all heavy smokers, will die of lung cancer. And none would state that cigarette smoking is the only thing that can cause lung cancer. These caveats do nothing to diminish the fact that cigarette smoking causes lung cancer.

During my pathology classes, I remember being impressed with the term "pathognomonic." The term means a sign or symptom that is so distinctive that it allows one to make a diagnosis of a specific disease. In all diseases, including infectious diseases, pathognomonic signs and symptoms are very rare. From my knowledge of viral diseases, only smallpox or measles come close in that all newly infected subjects who have never been exposed or vaccinated reveal a distinctive pattern of spots within a short period after exposure. More typical are viral infections like flu or COVID, where many show a serious systemic illness, some show nothing, and a few die. Or hepatitis B viruses, where many show nothing, some show severe systemic disease because of liver cell destruction, and a small fraction get lethal liver cancer. Or papilloma viruses, where most get nothing or a few warts, but some get lethal cancer of the uterine cervix or penis. To physicians and medical scientists, all of these viruses clearly cause disease.

Another important lesson I've learned from epidemiology is the value of prospective studies. In retrospective studies, it is often hard to control all the variables – for example, because the disease outcomes may be biased by the method the investigator used to collect the cases. With prospective studies, one can follow a cohort of homosexual men with seemingly equal characteristics, conduct an HIV test, and then follow both the infected and uninfected people for several years. If the HIV-positive people have more obvious decreases in immune lymphocytes, more illness, and more deaths following a statistical analysis of the data, it is easy to conclude that HIV is the cause of those outcomes. The only reasonable alternative explanation, it seems to me, is that HIV is a clear indicator for the outcomes, even though, at least theoretically, something else that causes AIDS may be activating HIV if the HIV isn't causing the pathology. Even that unlikely scenario can be tossed out for AIDS since the advent of effective drugs in the early to mid-1990s. Most of these drugs were designed to very specifically attack an essential viral enzyme that HIV needs to replicate. If you block the virus in this way, amounts of virus in the blood drop dramatically and rapidly, lymphocyte numbers rebound, and patients don't get sick or die. Such results were produced and reconfirmed by numerous researchers and clinicians by the mid- to late 1990s, yet Duesberg and his troupe would ignore such evidence and continue to spout their nonsense for at least another 15 years.

Duesberg first published an opinion piece about his denialism in 1987 in *Cancer Research*.[88,89] He followed this with letters to *Science* and *Nature*. One of his key arguments was that HIV couldn't cause AIDS because it took too long to develop, up to 10 years. In fact, many viruses cause diseases only after several years, some, like herpes zoster, causing shingles after several decades. When a group at Columbia University made the discovery of a new herpes virus that caused Kaposi sarcoma in 1994,[18] Duesberg argued that therefore HIV didn't cause AIDS because Kaposi sarcoma was AIDS. But just as HIV damages the immune system to allow the development of pneumonia from Pneumocystis or tuberculosis from bacteria, HIV created the immune system pathology that made all those infections more dangerous. One might be considered direct and one indirect, but it hardly matters which if the patient is so debilitated he cannot mount normal immune resistance.

Journalists and editors sometimes like to include dissidents such as Duesberg in their coverage, as an entertaining controversy may increase readership. John Maddox, the editor of *Nature,* took this approach in the mid-1990s when he seemed to encourage

Duesberg to write a dissenting letter in response to some recently published papers that illuminated how the destruction of lymphocytes occurs after HIV infection. But Duesberg's submission was so far from the reality of the actual data, Maddox decided he couldn't publish it. Duesberg then accused him of hypocrisy. Farhad Manjoo, an opinion columnist for the *New York Times*, recently wrote a piece that brilliantly summarizes my own position with respect to Duesberg and the denialists. In response to Rober F. Kennedy Jr.'s recent campaign against vaccines, he wrote that "the thing a conspiracy theorist desires most [is] recognition that his arguments are important enough to merit serious debate ... You can come armed with all the facts in the world, but when you're dealing with a conspiracist, there's no real way to 'win' an argument. For people whose views aren't anchored to facts, winning is simply getting attention – and when you publicly argue with someone like Kennedy, you've already lost."[90] Kellyanne Conway, describing some of Donald Trump's "alternative facts," is another illustration of the problem of dealing with conspiracists and denialists.

Duesberg also attracted a following of fellow denialists. One was Henry Bauer, a professor at Virginia Tech, who questioned whether HIV exists at all because the "tests are not accurate." Duesberg recognized the existence of HIV, just argued that it is harmless. Bauer was also known as a leader in the movement to accept the legitimacy of the Loch Ness monster. Another, Jad Adams, published a book entitled *AIDS: The HIV Myth,* which is largely devoted to the positions of Duesberg.[91] Another denialist was Matthias Rath, a vitamin salesman from Germany who claimed that his nutritional supplements could treat and cure diabetes, cardiovascular disease, cancer, and HIV/AIDS. An excellent book on these and other denialists was published by Seth Kalichman, a professor of social psychology at the University of Connecticut.[92] After the development of effective drugs against HIV in the 1990s, when AIDS was no longer a death sentence, the denialists' audience in the United States and Europe evaporated. But the denialists then turned their attention to Africa, where the effective drugs were generally unavailable because of their cost. The result would be catastrophic for the Republic of South Africa.

It is unclear, at least to me, how the president of South Africa, Thabo Mbeki, first connected with Duesberg. It happened in the late 1990s as the HIV epidemic was exploding in that country. He and some other African leaders had a natural tendency to minimize the AIDS epidemic because it scared away tourists. This had a damper effect on attempts to educate the population about unsafe sex and condom use. The new wave of very effective anti-HIV drugs would be expensive with millions infected, at least for the first few years of that epidemic. Mbeki did not recognize the importance of mother-to-child transmission of HIV by pregnant women and thus that AIDS in babies could be largely prevented at very low cost. He and his minister of health, Manto Tshabalala-Msimang, thought AIDS was just caused by poverty. Of course it is not, with some of the wealthiest countries in Africa and the world having the highest infection rates. But after the availability of effective drugs, poverty often did stand in the way of accessing the lifesaving treatment. Perhaps it shouldn't be surprising that Mbeki and Tshabalala-Msimang would find solace with Duesberg and his crew. Duesberg's friend Rath, the vitamin salesman, might naturally bond with Tshabalala-Msimang, as she was also known as "Dr. Beetroot" because she stated that beetroot, garlic, and African potatoes worked better for the treatment of AIDS than did drugs against HIV.

In the year 2000, Durban was selected as the site for the annual International AIDS Conference, which regularly drew many thousands of participants. In advance of the meeting, Mbeki organized his own advisory committee to inform his policy on AIDS. He insisted that the committee be comprised of equal numbers of those who believed HIV caused AIDS and denialists who did not. Duesberg and his following had the upper hand on the committee, encouraging policy recognizing that AIDS didn't exist and that the HIV drugs were harmful as well as costly. More than 5,000 AIDS scientists and physicians at the international conference, including myself, signed a declaration to refute Mbeki's pronouncements and policies. Later, Stephen Lewis, the United Nations special envoy for AIDS in Africa, stated publicly that South Africa promoted a "lunatic fringe" attitude toward HIV and AIDS, describing the government as "obtuse, dilatory, and negligent about rolling out treatment."[93] In about 2002, after much of the damage had already been done, Mbeki asked Duesberg and the denialists to stop associating his name with theirs.

Dr. Pride Chigwedere, a young physician and PhD student in my lab from Zimbabwe, became so upset with the Duesberg/Mbeki situation that he took time away from his successful lab work to focus on what he called "public health malpractice." He felt there had to be some disciplinary action against those who, like Duesberg, publicly advise the population against good health practices, and he published a paper on the subject.[94] It was a good idea, but I reluctantly advised him that enforcement would be near impossible as public health practitioners who are not physicians have no licenses or certifications that can be revoked in the event of malpractice, as do physicians involved in regular medical practice. He did, however, take classes in economics at Harvard and conduct an analysis of how many lives were lost in South Africa due to Mbeki's AIDS policies in the early years.[95] Using mathematical modeling, his best estimate was that 330,000 South African lives were lost because a feasible program with anti-HIV drugs was not implemented in the period 2000–2005. It was estimated that 35,000 infants became infected because the simple and inexpensive mother-to-child transmission prophylaxis program with nevirapine was not implemented.[95]

Duesberg responded with his usual arguments – that the drugs didn't inhibit HIV and that HIV was harmless. His paper, which had already been rejected by the *Journal of Acquired Immune Deficiency Syndromes*, a standard AIDS journal, was then published by *Medical Hypotheses*, a journal that was intended as a forum for unconventional ideas without the traditional filter of scientific peer review. The publisher, Elsevier, was embarrassed by the decision and withdrew the paper after 13 of the 19 editorial board members wrote to protest the decision by the editor to publish the paper. At about the same time, a large number of AIDS researchers contacted the National Library of Medicine to ask that *Medical Hypotheses* be dropped from the Medline and PubMed databases. The editor of the journal was subsequently sacked.

By this time, about 2010, many millions of lives of AIDS patients had been saved by the use of anti-HIV drugs and many other HIV infections prevented as the drugs rendered those who were already infected much less infectious to others. Duesberg wasn't quite ready to stop his shenanigans, however, as he found an obscure Italian journal to publish his paper.[96] That, too, resulted in resignations and unrest on the editorial board of the *Italian Journal of Anatomy and Embryology*.

We can hope that the chances for Duesberg and his group to have much impact from their messages of public health malpractice is finished. However, public health quackery and the popularization of pseudoscience on other matters is still in place. Through his anti-vaccine movement, spreading misinformation and propaganda, Robert F. Kennedy Jr. could eventually do even more harm than Duesberg. Building on a fraudulent paper that claimed a link between vaccines and autism,[97] Kennedy has revitalized a cadre of vaccine denialists who, together, may cause many innocent people to ignore the tremendous benefits of most vaccines. If their pseudoscience campaigns are effective, it endangers not just their own followers but many others as it interferes with the chances to reach effective "herd immunity" to reduce transmissions through the multiplier effect.

chapter fourteen

Why No Vaccine?

In 1984, Secretary of Health and Human Services Margaret Heckler called a press conference with Dr. Bob Gallo to announce that Gallo's group at the National Institutes of Health (NIH) had found the cause of AIDS, a retrovirus that would later be renamed the human immunodeficiency virus (HIV). They also mentioned that a vaccine for HIV might be tested in about 2 years. For many who listened, including AIDS researchers such as myself, this seemed optimistic. But most of us probably did expect that we would have a vaccine within 10–15 years. In retrospect, we were all wrong. Now, about 40 years later, no HIV vaccine product is even on the horizon.

Indeed, it is questionable whether we now even need an HIV vaccine. Not because HIV or AIDS disease has gone away. It hasn't. HIV infections will probably be with us for the next 50 years or more.

Two exploratory trials for an HIV vaccine did begin within a few years after the press conference. But both were in people who were already infected with HIV. Thus, the vaccines were really putative therapeutic interventions to determine if the health of the AIDS patients could be improved by further stimulating immunity. Almost all existing vaccines, except perhaps rabies, are to prevent or attenuate an initial infection, not to treat an infection that is already present. One of these trials was conducted by a French investigator Dr. Daniel Zagury in collaboration with Congolese investigators. Zagury injected himself and also a few AIDS patients in Kinshasa, Zaire, with a bioengineered preparation. Dr. Robert Redfield, who was recently head of the US Centers for Disease

Control and Prevention (CDC), also led a small trial in the United States using a different bioengineered product. At that time, Redfield was a military physician, and the volunteers were members of the US Army. The results of both trials were controversial.[98] Few physicians believed, either then or now, that any vaccine had much of a chance if used in HIV/AIDS patients. But testing anything in patients who are likely to die soon, as AIDS patients were then, is usually much easier for ethical reasons. As with terminal cancer patients, untested interventions with any hope of benefit are often tested under a rationale of compassion.

At the time of the Heckler press conference, there was no mention of making drugs to save the lives of AIDS patients who were already infected. The development of antiviral drugs, unlike the situation with antibacterial drugs or antibiotics, was in its infancy. Drugs to treat most viral diseases were then considered unrealistic or impossible. Ironically, the reason a vaccine for HIV may no longer be needed is because drugs were developed, and they were eventually proven to be very effective. Such AIDS drugs are now used routinely to save lives and restore health to HIV-infected people. They can also be used to prevent infection if taken prophylactically. And when infected people are given the right drugs, they are no longer infectious for others. The first and second generations of drugs were less effective and had serious side effects, causing patients to interrupt treatment and generate more drug-resistant variants. The current generation of anti-HIV drugs has no such problems, so they may be taken for life. With the slow-release forms of administration, the drugs might be taken only once per month and probably even less often in the future.

Most vaccines are made by pharmaceutical or biotechnology companies who are driven by market opportunities. Vaccines are rarely moneymakers, unless the government is paying for both the cost of development and purchasing the vaccine. Conversely, drugs for common problems like hypertension, depression, or diabetes may be very profitable, especially if large fractions of rich Western populations are on the drugs for much of their adult lives. Drugs for AIDS may be a major product if millions are taking them for life after an initial diagnosis in their 20s or 30s.

Vaccines may also be even more expensive to develop than drugs, especially if one considers the immense cost of efficacy trials. Furthermore, the widespread availability of good drugs for HIV/AIDS has probably made the cost of testing an HIV vaccine even more expensive and perhaps impossible without large governmental financing – assuming adherence to acceptable standards for human subjects experimentation. The first stage of testing is done using low doses of the candidate vaccine and only a few dozen volunteers, with an equal or almost equal number of volunteers getting a placebo control. For all trials that would ultimately be acceptable for US Food and Drug Administration (FDA) approval, the trials would be randomized for vaccine versus placebo and double blind so that neither the participants nor the physician would know whether they received vaccine or placebo. The trial participants would all be monitored frequently for a year or so to verify that the experimental vaccine did not produce any toxicity or harmful effects. The main goal for the first phase is to confirm that the vaccine is safe. If there are no toxic side effects, a phase II trial could then begin. It would be an expanded study on safety, again with randomization including placebo controls and double blinded. For phase II, however, multiple graduated doses might be used, and a few hundred participants would be enrolled. Along with all the checks for toxic side effects, immune responses of the subjects would be checked to see if the vaccine elicits meaningful levels of immune antibodies. If the vaccine works well, it would be both safe, with no appreciable side effects, and it would produce high levels of antibodies as an indication of good immunogenicity. Probably more than 100 vaccines have already been tested for HIV in more than 200 phase I and/or phase II trials. Almost all experimental vaccines tested appeared safe, but almost all were insufficiently immunogenic, unable to induce levels of antibodies that were thought necessary to be protective. So the candidate vaccines were dropped and deemed inappropriate to justify testing in a phase III trial.

For the few experimental vaccines that might advance to phase III trials based on a safe profile and an indication of a strong immune stimulation effect or immunogenicity, a much larger phase III trial might be planned. This would include many more people, probably thousands of subjects, selected for their high likelihood of being naturally exposed to HIV. The volunteer subjects are again randomized to receive either the vaccine or a placebo, with a double blinded design so the enrollees wouldn't tend to alter their HIV exposure risk according to whether they received the vaccine or the placebo. The size of the trial is based on the best estimate of the number of volunteers that would have to be enrolled to show a statistically significant difference in the outcomes. Those who received the vaccine would have to show a lower rate of HIV infection than those who received the placebo, with the difference being great enough that it would not have occurred due to chance alone.

To meet ethical requirements, all volunteer participants should receive intensive education to avoid exposure to HIV, such as by unsafe sexual practices, even though this may increase the numbers of enrollees that would be needed. As the incidence of new infections gets lower, whether by education or any other means, the larger the number of enrollees needed to have enough new HIV infections to see a statistically significant difference between those who received vaccine versus placebo. So the trial design experts would inevitably look to involve populations with the highest risk for HIV infection. In the era when most experimental vaccine designs might be ready for testing, by the early years of the 2000s, these populations might be homosexual men in the United States or Europe, or young sexually active heterosexuals in Africa.

As the burden of AIDS became much greater in Africa, both because of higher incidence and because of lower access to expensive drugs for treatment, it was clearly logical to design, test, and ultimately use any successful vaccine in the African populations where it was most needed. But this also raised concerns among Africans that they might be used as "guinea pigs" to make a vaccine product that might not be available to them if the costs were too high, as they clearly were at that time for the best AIDS drugs.

Our research group at Harvard was one of many that had an interest in making a vaccine for HIV/AIDS. We had discovered the HIV molecules, gp120 and gp160, that were widely believed to be the most important ingredient of a vaccine.[70] We also invested substantial time investigating why these molecules should be the most effective viral stimulant of the immune response[73] and in characterizing which types of immune responses might be most important to induce. These obviously included antibodies[72] but also cell-mediated responses whereby killer T lymphocytes are induced to attack HIV-infected cells.[99] We even designed a new hybrid virus made using HIV and a related monkey virus we had identified earlier.[100] This could then be used to test HIV vaccine candidates in monkeys before trying them in people.

Ironically, we also had experience making the only currently available vaccine against a virus like HIV. This was the feline retrovirus that causes immunosuppression and leukemia in cats.[101] This helped establish the belief that vaccines could be made against viruses that infect lymphocytes, even against viruses that integrate their own genome into the host cellular DNA. Unfortunately, the cat virus system did not give us important information about the problem of extreme mutational change that is the hallmark of HIV. While seen to some extent with flu viruses, HIV undergoes constant change in infected people. That explains why a newly infecting HIV will always be different from the HIV represented in the vaccine. It also explains why drug resistance happens so fast, especially if the patient received only one drug, like AZT, at a time.

As designing a vaccine is a major scientific undertaking, preparing for trials is also a major diplomatic challenge. If a quarter or more of the general population is afraid of already existing proven vaccines, we can only imagine how many people might be afraid of unproven experimental vaccines. In the early 1980s, I was a volunteer in a small vaccine trial for hepatitis B virus. Of 16 of us who volunteered, I was 1 of only 3 or 4 who had no side effects. Although the side effects were mild and temporary, they created even more apprehension for future enrollees. That vaccine was subsequently modified to be very safe, and it was highly efficacious in protecting against infection with hepatitis B virus.

While seeking to test an HIV vaccine that would be appropriate for southern Africa, we had numerous consultations with community and national leaders in Botswana. A community advisory board was established. It included local leaders of medical

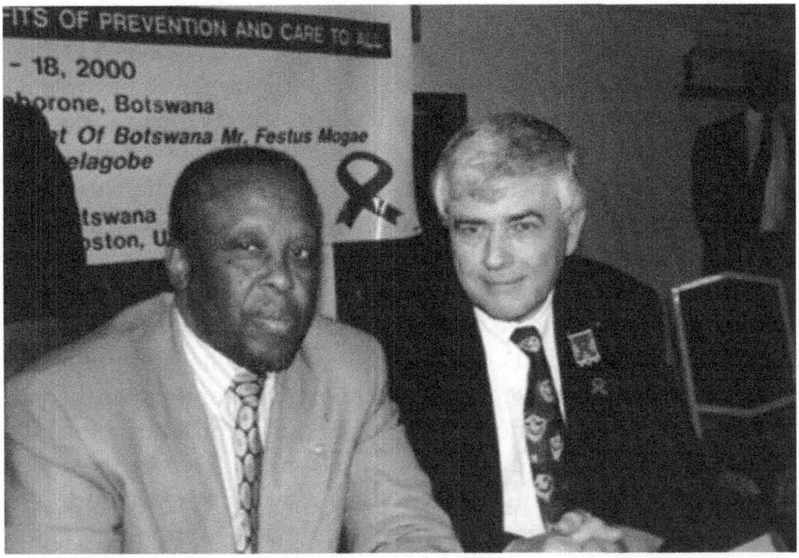

Figure 14.1: President Festus Mogae, Max Essex

services, educational institutions, businesses, and the clergy. They met monthly with me or another member of our research team. We explained our goals for testing a vaccine and how and why the vaccine was made. We took questions, and the group would then discuss concerns and issues without us, with any further questions to be raised at the next meeting. We had similar meetings with members of Parliament and tribal chiefs. On one occasion, President Mogae called a meeting of senior health advisors for a similar briefing and mentioned his support.

We still anticipated that it might be difficult to find a sufficient number of volunteers to fulfill the trial requirements until we could establish a bond of trust. Reverend Rupert Hambira, who was president of the Council of Churches in Botswana, then invited me to raise the vaccine trial issue at a church service. It was the largest congregation in the capital city, with several hundred in attendance. I spoke for about 10 minutes about HIV/AIDS, the need for a vaccine, and the need for trial volunteers. Most of the congregants had been there many times before to attend funerals of AIDS patients.[102] As soon as I finished speaking, Reverend Hambira asked for questions. One of the first to raise her hand was an elderly woman whom I recognized. She was Lady Masire, the wife of the last president of the country, Quett Masire. She commented only to say that she knew me and that the citizens could trust us. It was spontaneous and very effective. We began the trial soon after and had more volunteers than we could enroll.

Most vaccines that are currently used in people are safe and remarkably cost effective as they prevent more severe diseases in both children and adults. Measles, mumps, rubella, and polio vaccines are made from live viruses that were deliberately weakened. A live weakened vaccine was never seriously considered for HIV because the virus could still insert itself in the DNA of the vaccinated person, and it might revert to full virulence with more replication. Flu vaccine has generally been made from whole killed virus grown in chicken eggs. It is somewhat less protective than the others because flu viruses often change their surface proteins through mutation, though not at the extremely high level seen with HIV. Hepatitis B and shingles vaccines are bioengineered subunits, similar to most HIV experimental vaccine designs. However, they are highly immunogenic and much more effective than the HIV candidate vaccines tested thus far. The recent COVID vaccines represent a giant leap forward in the science of vaccinology. Made from pieces of RNA to mimic genes of the virus, they are remarkably immunogenic and safe. Unfortunately, this new technology is not likely to solve the inherent problems in making an HIV vaccine. The greatest of these is the extremely rapid mutational changes associated with HIV, which cannot be overcome with the new RNA vaccines.

One of the greatest accomplishments of public health practice was the worldwide eradication of smallpox, which happened about 45 years ago. It was achieved because of the availability of an effective and inexpensive vaccine. People who were infected could be readily identified by their pox spots, and teams of physicians supported by the World Health Organization (WHO) and the CDC were used throughout the world to administer the vaccine.

Wherever a case was found, a team would go and vaccinate everyone around the case who could possibly have contact with infected people. Political cooperation and diplomacy were certainly as important as the vaccine. Societal and political cooperation have recently deteriorated at both the national and international levels, so making any new efforts at disease eradication through vaccination seems futile. It has been estimated that death rates from COVID were 43% higher for Republicans in Florida and Ohio in association with lower vaccination rates.[103] We can only imagine how many lives will be lost if many people listen to Robert F. Kennedy Jr., the anti-vax conspiracist politician.

COVID, flu, and most other vaccines are not capable of inducing sterilizing immunity. Sterilizing immunity is where the protection is so perfect that the infecting virus cannot replicate at all in the exposed person. The more common situation, as with COVID, is that the vaccine can only induce non-sterilizing immunity. After vaccination, the person still gets infected if exposed to the virus, but the infection is attenuated, avoiding severe disease and hospitalization. Only small amounts of virus can replicate, and those small amounts are too little to cause disease. This is a satisfactory situation for most viral vaccines, but not for HIV because any HIV replication results in permanent latent infection in the host cell DNA. This is an additional reason why an ideal vaccine for HIV is almost impossible to imagine. Fortunately, because of the great drugs now available, we probably don't even need one.

As I began to appreciate the dilemma of trying to make an HIV vaccine, I was again impressed by how unprecedented the AIDS epidemic and its origin really were. By comparison, the COVID epidemic seems somewhat easier to explain. The origins of COVID and HIV are covered in the next two chapters.

chapter fifteen

The Origin of Viral Epidemics 101 – COVID

Most new epidemics in people begin when a virus from a lower animal species enters the human population. Diseases transmitted from animals to people are called zoonoses. Some, like rabies, occur via a rare bite from a rabid dog, raccoon, or bat. But the rabid person, once infected, is a "dead-end host," assuming that person doesn't bite another person. For many other zoonotic viruses, like the COVIDs or flu, expansion of the viral pathogen first occurs in an intermediate "amplifier" host before expansion as an epidemic in people.

Loony conspiracists seem to be having a heyday with our current COVID epidemic. Some, like David Icke and Alex Jones, claim that the COVID epidemic doesn't exist, a position that might make Peter Duesberg proud. Others agree that the epidemic does exist but believe it was caused by the 5G network or by genetically modified crops. Some want to believe that the recent COVID epidemic began with Chinese virologists deliberately making a designer virus, using US money from Dr. Tony Fauci to wreak havoc on the world. Truth and knowledge don't seem to count for much in politics these days. But we must make them count in medicine, epidemiology, and public health if we want to stay alive.

To understand the origin of our current COVID epidemic, and whether it came from a research lab or a "wet market" in Wuhan, China, one must first recognize that we've had at least three different new COVID epidemics in the last 20 years. It is highly likely that we've had more than three. It seems possible, even likely, that some smaller epidemics could have emerged in regions of the world where people eat wild animals or have exposure to bats.

The first of the three well characterized COVID epidemics was called SARS-1. SARS stands for "severe acute respiratory syndrome." It could have been called COVID-1, except that we didn't know it was caused by a coronavirus when it first emerged. SARS-1 surfaced in 2003 and was of most concern in Hong Kong, Singapore, and Toronto.[104] It caused fear and panic because the mortality rate was high, about 10%.

In 2008, Dr. Yichen Lu of my research group and I edited a book entitled *Emerging Infections in Asia*.[105] The book had a section entitled "SARS." It had chapters on SARS-1 in China, Singapore, and Taiwan. Yichen was from mainland China and had conducted research there on HIV and tuberculosis. An author of one chapter on SARS-1 in China was Dr. Li Ruan, who also spent time in our lab and then returned to the Chinese CDC. The author of the chapter on Taiwan was Dr. Yi-Ming Chen, a professor at Kaohsiung Medical University, who was a research doctoral student with me about 30 years ago. The author of another chapter was Dr. Zhengli Shi, who did pioneering studies on the origin of the coronavirus that caused SARS-1.[4] Her work was important for understanding the origin of the current COVID epidemic of 2019–2023.

Dr. Shi's group initially suggested that a likely origin for SARS-1 was the masked palm civet, a raccoon-like mammal found in China and other countries in the region. After the wild-caught animals became a delicacy in wet markets, farmers began to breed them in captivity to increase the numbers available to eat. In an initial survey of animals from a live-animal market in Guangdong Province, four of six masked palm civets were positive for a virus that was very closely related, if not identical, to the coronavirus of SARS-1. A similar virus was found in a raccoon dog. Antibodies to the SARS-1 virus were found in about one-third of people (11 of 35) who were wild animal traders or butchers in the market. In another survey of 508 animal traders from three animal markets in Guangdong Province, 66 (13%) were positive for COVID antibodies.[106] The highest rates of antibodies (73%) were found in those who sold masked palm civets. Those who traded in cats, snakes, or fowl had much lower rates of antibodies. Another research group looked at traders who sold only masked palm civets and found 59% (24 of 41) positive. In a control group of 139 traders who only handled vegetables, 1 was positive. Taken at face value, these results obviously suggest that viruses from masked palm civets might have infected many people in the wet markets. Remarkably, the complete gene sequence of two civet isolates were more than 99% identical to a human isolate.[107]

Masked palm civets in the wild are solitary and nocturnal, making them hard to study before being caught in traps. However, it has been estimated that there were about 40,000 palm civets being raised in about 600 farms in 2003, when the epidemic started. By 2004, after being linked with SARS, many of them were eliminated.

Recognizing that many viruses are present in bats, Chinese investigators also checked various species of bats from Guangxi, Guangdong, and Hong Kong.[4] A third or more of the bats were positive for either SARS-related antibodies or related viral genome sequences. The highest rates were in horseshoe bats. Although the bats themselves may be eaten by people in Africa and Asia, that is probably unusual in this region of China.

In summary, it is not necessary to believe that COVID came from a lab-made virus or even an accidental virus release for SARS-1. To me, it seems just as likely that the virus came from a wet-market animal handler via civets or a related species. The civets probably became infected from horseshoe bats, and the civets functioned as an amplifier host who had more contact with people. It is also possible that the SARS-1 could have come directly to people from bats.

The second recent epidemic of coronaviruses in people was identified in 2012. It appeared to have nothing to do with either civets or China. It developed in the Middle East, first recognized in Saudi Arabia, clearly having something to do with camels. Some people apparently kiss their camels, and the animals are sometimes also butchered for meat. Most people in the United States or Europe aren't even aware of this epidemic. It was usually called MERS for "Middle East respiratory syndrome."[108] The nomenclature may be confusing. The recognition of MERS means that our current COVID epidemic (2019–2023) is actually the third recent coronavirus epidemic, even though it has also been called SARS-CoV-2 as well as COVID-19.

Taken at face value, the Middle East would seem like an odd place for a new epidemic of respiratory disease to arise. Flu and other respiratory viruses get transmitted best in cold, humid environments with high population density. Saudi Arabia doesn't seem to fit.

I had an interesting trip to Riyadh in the early 1990s, after being invited to lecture on HIV/AIDS and to consult with the minister of health. The invitation included a first-class ticket on Saudia Airlines. Before dinner on the plane, the server appeared with a large bowl of beluga caviar, offering ice cream scoop size portions, but of course no alcohol. Upon arrival, I was taken to a luxury hotel and put up in a six-room suite that included a formal dining room and a library. As I walked away from the podium after lecturing, the moderator slipped me an envelope. I was pleasantly surprised to discover that it contained a thick wad of $100 bills. It was a gift. I hadn't asked for a fee. I can see why the professional golfers and Jared Kushner wanted to do business there. Along with a few colleagues, I was then taken for a traditional dinner of barbecued sheep, falafel, and tabouli that took place several miles out in the Arabian desert. Camels were part of the travel entourage. I did see facial contact between the camels, but not between camels and their drivers, and camel meat was not on the dinner menu.

MERS has a mortality rate over 30%, considerably higher than COVID-19, where it is 2% or less, or even SARS-1 at 10%. Patients with MERS have essentially the same symptoms as those with COVID-19 or SARS-1, especially fever and respiratory difficulties, but for MERS the symptoms are usually more severe. A large fraction of MERS patients also had kidney disease, whereas most patients with SARS-1 or COVID-19 do not.[109]

MERS has received less attention because only a few thousand cases have been documented, as opposed to hundreds of millions of people who have had COVID-19. With MERS, it seems that people are more often infected directly from camels than from other people, though person-to-person transmission also occurs. Bats are again thought to play an important role for MERS by infecting the camels. It is recommended that people who are around camels, especially in the Middle East, should wear masks to avoid infection with the coronavirus of MERS. Our current pandemic of COVID-19 is the third epidemic of the last 20 years, but obviously more expansive and durable than the first two. COVID-19 has had a significantly lower mortality rate, but with hundreds of millions of infections, it has already resulted in 4–5 million deaths. The earliest reactions by Republican politicians in the United States seem to have been to play down general strategies to prevent infections, such as closing schools, discouraging large indoor events, and wearing masks. Later, as vaccines became available, some of the same conservative leaders would minimize their effects. Most vaccines, including those for COVID, do not completely prevent infection. They do, however, restrict the ability of the virus to replicate to a level required to cause disease signs and symptoms or death. So fully vaccinated people are more likely to get only a mild "common cold" type of response. Vaccination will also make infected people much less likely to transmit to others.

In a recent article, David Quammen presented an analysis of theories about the origin of the virus that caused the current COVID-19 pandemic.[110] One theory, and certainly the one I favor, is that the initial COVID-19 virus entered the human population through some wet-market type of association with animals like civets or perhaps a raccoon dog in this case.

The second alternative theory is that the COVID-19 virus started as a laboratory "leak," where personnel at the Wuhan Institute of Virology accidentally got infected and in turn infected others outside the lab. This is reasonable to imagine, as the lab of Dr. Zhengli Shi had been studying bat and wet-market-type viruses since the first recent COVID virus outbreak, SARS-1, in 2003.[4] Viruses from bats, other animals, and SARS-1-infected people were all maintained in that lab to study similarities and differences. To analyze the viruses in detail, they are often concentrated to unnatural levels, and some of the lab procedures might include the unintentional production of aerosols. Because concentrated viruses pose obvious risks for the laboratory workers, such procedures are normally done in highly regulated facilities deliberately designed for such work. These include negative-pressure rooms and hoods to pull out aerosolized fluids and gases to protect the personnel. But accidents can happen. It just seems to me that the overwhelming evidence that numerous COVID infections seemed to occur around SARS-1 wet-market workers, based on the fact that half or more had antibodies,[106] as did many camel trainers for MERS, makes the market exposure for COVID-19 much more likely than a lab release.

The third hypothesis about the potential origin for COVID-19 is that the current virus was designed in the lab as a bioweapon.[111] This seems very unlikely to me. While it is possible to genetically engineer a virus to have greater ability to infect and/or kill human cells in the lab, such designed characteristics would almost surely not translate into what COVID-19 did in a population of people. Human bodily defenses are astoundingly complicated, and the genetic variation of potential immune responses among people is almost unlimited. The endless natural generation of viruses in bats and amplifier animals in the market makes it far more likely that a virus evolving in that milieu would have the right stuff, and the wet-market employees would provide many more opportunities than the lab workers. No serious scientist has argued that SARS-1 or MERS were purposefully created in a lab, and certainly no one could argue that the various human coronaviruses of the "common cold," in people long before SARS-1 or even before lab virologists could do genetic engineering, were of lab origin.

Regardless of the biological or evolutionary origin of the COVID-19 virus, the epidemic was more severe than it needed to be. Effective vaccines were produced much more rapidly than most of us would have predicted. But conspiracies, disinformation, and partisan politics prevented the rapid development of effective public health policy. The result was more disease and death along with more severe damage to the economy.

A recent opinion piece in the *Washington Post* pointed out how Chinese physicians, public health officials, and scientists have been gagged and dissuaded from cooperating with Western scientists or the World Health Organization.[112] This is an unfortunate response by the Chinese political leaders, which makes things worse. But before the politicization of COVID-19 in early 2020, Chinese scientists we've had contact with, including Zhengli Shi in Wuhan, had been very cooperative. At this point, it is almost certain that we'll never know for sure where the virus came from, but natural evolution through bats and wet-market animals is certainly the best bet.

Most, but not all, new or newly identified epidemics are caused by viruses. Most that are seen for the first time in people originate from wild animal species, often rodents, bats, or birds. Climate change, changes in agricultural practices, and movement of human populations associated with economic, social, and political pressures can all result in the development and expansion of epidemics. Two new epidemics of the last century, HIV/AIDS and COVID, have killed millions as they rapidly expanded to become pandemics. Despite the best efforts of scientists, physicians, and public health experts, both were then associated with political and social upheavals.

chapter sixteen

The Origin of Viral Epidemics 102 – HIVs

As with the coronaviruses, it seems clear that the HIVs of AIDS have entered the human population quite a few different times. In the case of HIV, the site of entry was tropical Africa, not Asia, and the animal host source was nonhuman primates, not civets or raccoon dogs or bats. The significance of wet markets may be equally appropriate – in the HIV case, the butchering of chimpanzees and monkeys. The most important entry that could be deduced for HIV-1 may have occurred about a hundred years ago in the region of southern Cameroon or the former Belgian Congo.

The HIV-1 of the current pandemic that has infected approximately 100 million people and killed an estimated 40 million almost certainly came in from a chimp. The initial mortality in people was near 100%, but the patients took 5–10 years to die, so there was ample opportunity for transmission. At least three additional entries of HIV-1s to people have occurred from either chimps or gorillas, but none of these have apparently spread to more than 100,000 people. The most successful entrant gave rise to the group called M, for main or major, which soon gave rise to more than a dozen distinct subtypes that then circulated in human populations in different regions of the world.

The HIV-2s, first identified by our research team on the basis of cross-reactivity with monkey viruses, apparently entered people from monkeys first in West Africa, around the region of Guinea-Bissau.[113] Multiple entries of different groups and subtypes of HIV-2 have also occurred in West Africa. HIV-2 was shown to be

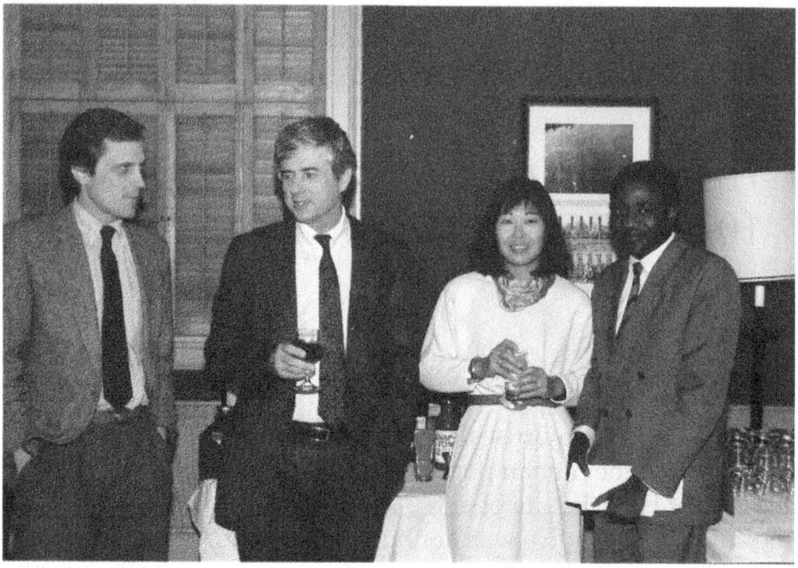

Figure 16.1: Ric Marlink, Max Essex, Phyllis Kanki, Souleymane Mboup

less transmissible by Drs. Phyllis Kanki and Richard Marlink of our group, helping to explain why there has been very limited spread throughout the world.[84] Nonetheless, we can estimate that HIV-2 has infected at least several million people and killed at least one-quarter or one-third of them.

The virus that has been responsible for almost all infections in the United States and Western Europe, as well as much of South America and Asia, is the HIV-1 group M subtype B. It was also the first HIV detected in Africa. In a collaboration with Dr. Andre Nahmias and his research group at Emory University in Atlanta, we examined 672 stored human samples from Kisangani and Kinshasa, collected in the late 1950s, in what was then the Belgian Congo.[114] One person was clearly positive. A later study by others using polymerase chain reaction (PCR) showed that the plasma from this person contained remnants of the HIV-1B subtype genome.[115] Surprisingly, numerous studies on human samples from various places in sub-Saharan Africa collected 20–30 years later showed that B had essentially disappeared but had been replaced by other subtypes, especially HIV-1 subtypes A, C, and D. Why this happened is a mystery, especially when recognizing that the epidemics in the United States and Western Europe were, and still are, subtype B.

The Democratic Republic of Congo (DRC), formerly called Belgian Congo and Zaire, is an interesting place. Beginning in 1986, I traveled to the DRC on several occasions to arrange collaborations and establish partnerships with colleagues in Kinshasa, the capital, and Lubumbashi, the largest city in the southeastern part of the country. We began to do joint studies with Dr. Raphael Kalengayi, who was head of pathology at the University of Kinshasa, and with Dr. Lukumuena Oscar Kashala, a young associate of Kalengayi who would subsequently spend time with us in Boston completing a PhD degree at Harvard. Even the government seemed cooperative, despite the rampant poverty. The Minister of Health hosted a reception for us at a governmental parlor, bringing together leaders in the medical area. We were served fine cognac from France and Oreo cookies from the United States. We had been told in advance that wearing neckties was illegal.

We then moved on to Lubumbashi, chosen because it is the home base of Gécamines, one of the largest mining companies in Africa with what seemed to be the most modern medical facilities in the country. We were successful in negotiating access to samples from hospital patients. We were then treated to dried caterpillars and beer at the home of a friend, and we went on to the local airport. I checked in for one night at a small local hotel called the Hilton. I showed the desk agent my card as a frequent Hilton Honors participant. He laughed and said, "We're not related to that Hilton." The next morning I flew to Kinshasa, then transferred to an Air Zaire flight destined for Brussels, with no X-ray screening at either Congolese airport.

After about 1960, when the Belgians left, there was massive expansion of cities like Kinshasa and Kisangani. With disproportionate numbers of young men, there was also a major expansion of female sex workers and sexually transmitted diseases. Many of the foreigners who worked at skilled jobs in Congo in the 1960s and

1970s were Haitian. This could help explain how Haiti became an early "hot spot" for HIV-1B in North America. Haiti also became a popular destination for "sex tourism," particularly for homosexual men from the United States. Dr. Jacques Pepin wrote an excellent book on potential routes for the early dissemination of HIV within and from Africa.[116] Regardless of how it happened, it seems surprising that the HIV epidemic in Africa is primarily due to heterosexual transmission, whereas the epidemic in the United States and Europe is primarily in male homosexuals and injection drug users. There is little evidence that HIV-1 subtype B still exists in sub-Saharan Africa, and none of the HIV-1 viruses that caused the massive heterosexual epidemics in Africa seemed to have taken hold in the United States or Europe.[117]

Soon after the HIVs were shown to have originated in African apes and monkeys, a theory surfaced speculating that the AIDS epidemic in Africa could have happened through the use of HIV-contaminated polio vaccines.[116] The supposed medical research culprit was Dr. Hilary Koprowski, a brilliant scientist and a friend. He did make one of the first oral polio vaccines, then in Poland, at about the same time that Dr. Albert Sabin did the same thing in the United States. But large trials with the same experimental vaccine were also done in Poland, where Koprowski lived at that time, but no HIV then surfaced in Poland. This did not stop the conspiracists from spinning the theory for political advantage. Among the conspiracists was Dr. Manto Tshabalala-Msimang, the health minister of South Africa from 1999 to 2007. She endorsed the theory while also still claiming that HIV was harmless.

Epidemiologists in the business of predicting the size and scope of an infectious disease epidemic usually think in terms of the reproduction number, designated as R_0. It refers to the contagiousness of a virus, like HIV or COVID, for a given population. The R_0 number is based on the average number of new people who become infected by an existing case. If the number is more than 1, the epidemic will expand. If below 1, the epidemic will eventually die out. But if an infected person remains contagious for many years, as do most HIV-1-infected people in the absence of good treatment, the epidemic may continue for many years. The higher the number is above 1, the faster the epidemic will spread. The R_0 number is particularly dependent on how many susceptible people are in the population, the contact rate, and the level of infectiousness – how much virus is released by each infected person – to determine the R_0. So the R_0 was much higher than 1 for the HIV-1 epidemic in sub-Saharan Africa in the late twentieth century and for COVID in most of the world in 2020 and 2021. The goal of "herd immunity" for COVID was sought by public health officials through high rates of vaccination to decrease the number of people who would be susceptible to COVID, thereby reducing the R_0 below 1.

With HIV-1, some believe that another variable called the "founder effect" may have played a role in the expansion of new epidemics of different HIV types or subtypes. In the United States and Western Europe, the HIV-1B expanded very rapidly in the highly susceptible subset of homosexual men who frequented bathhouses and practiced anal sex. Some argued that new HIV-1 subtypes that expanded so rapidly in Africa could not take hold because the most susceptible population, needed for introduction, was already saturated. A theoretical rationale for this could be based on our studies in West Africa showing that sex workers already infected with HIV-2 were less likely to get infected with HIV-1.[86]

The other sub-epidemics that happened early on in the United States and Europe were based on the rapid spread of HIV-1B in injection drug users. Because the optimal target cell for HIV infection is lymphocytes of the blood and lymph nodes, it can be assumed that all HIVs can spread with very high efficiency through blood transfusions.[118] The repeated use of contaminated needles by injection drug users (IDUs) or the use of HIV-contaminated blood clotting factors by hemophiliacs can be thought of as "mini-transfusions." In the case of IDU epidemics, politicians often interfered with good public health practice by blocking the distribution of clean needles.

As new and different HIV-1 subtypes moved around sub-Saharan Africa through heterosexual intercourse, different epidemics emerged. In the 1980s and early 1990s, the epidemic was a combination of HIV-1A and HIV-1D. It was particularly severe in Uganda and the countries around that region of East Africa like Kenya, Rwanda, and Burundi. As time went on, the epidemic moved southeast, especially documented by truck stops along the transit route from Kampala, Uganda, through Nairobi, Kenya, to Dar es Salaam in Tanzania. Later, in the 1990s, another even more explosive epidemic began in southeastern DRC and moved through Zambia and Malawi into most of the countries of southern Africa. The Republic of South Africa would soon have the largest number of HIV infections in the world. This epidemic was caused by HIV-1C, which seemed even more transmissible than the others.[76] In some countries, one-third or more of sexually active young women soon became infected.

It then became apparent to us that Tanzania was becoming a melting pot for the potential mixing of HIV-1s from the convergent movement of different epidemics. HIV-1A and HIV-1D viruses had recently moved in from Kenya and Uganda in the north, as the rapidly spreading HIV-1C began to move in from the epidemic in southern Africa. This seemed to present an unusual opportunity to see the rapid emergence of new hybrid viruses and the subsequent evolution and survival of any new viruses that had a selective fitness advantage. At the level of the viral genes, this is called recombination, because part of one viral parent, such as HIV-1A, could fuse with part of another viral parent, say an HIV-1C, to create a recombinant progeny virus called HIV-1A/C. If the virus is sufficiently viable to infect others, it would then become a circulating recombinant form (CRF) type of virus. This seemed important to understand because at least two new HIV-1 epidemics could be linked to CRF-type viruses rather than the conventional subtypes like A or C. One was a new and rapidly expanding epidemic in Thailand that was caused by the CRF virus HIV-1A/E, where an HIV-1A virus from East Africa somehow recombined with an HIV-1E virus from Central Africa and the progeny virus found its way to Asia. A second CRF virus, formed between HIV-1A and HIV-1G, was responsible for most of the new epidemic in West Africa. Even some of the pure subtypes seemed to evolve, as HIV-1D became less transmissible but more lethal than HIV-1A.

We began studying viruses in the Dar es Salaam and Kilimanjaro regions through a collaboration with Drs. Wafaie Fawzi and Saidi Kapiga, epidemiologists at Harvard who had a large nutrition project there. The people in Tanzania, although very poor, were knowledgeable about HIV/AIDS and cooperative with us. I recall relaxing evenings with Saidi and Dr. John Shao, the director of the Kilimanjaro Christian Medical Center, where we would sit in an outdoor restaurant below the snow-covered Kilimanjaro mountain discussing research plans. Ultimately, we examined new viruses from women who were hotel or bar workers in the region, as well as viruses from maternally infected newborn children. A large number of new hybrid viruses were found.[119] Their presence in newborns indicated that they had potential for spreading in the population with a possibility of causing new epidemics. Future studies in the region would be needed to determine which particular viral hybrids would be most likely to cause new epidemics.

The situation of the creation of new hybrid HIVs and their potential for future epidemics is reminiscent of influenza. For flu, new virus recombinants are generated, especially in wild birds in Asia. Each year, an international committee then recommends which variants should be selected for representation in the newest flu vaccine. The process is imperfect, which is why many flu vaccines offer only modest protection. For HIVs, the vaccine inclusion questions are not important as we have no vaccine. However, they may be important for detecting new HIV epidemics and potential resistance related to antiviral drugs used for treatment of HIV/AIDS.

chapter seventeen

Advances in Therapy

My introduction to viruses happened about 60 years ago in the 1960s. At that time, virologists had few tools with which to do experiments. One was to look at the viruses with an electron microscope. Even that approach was relatively new, and the very few microbiologists who had such an expensive instrument liked to show them off. As I was visiting scientists in various labs at the beginning of my career, I remember my wife Elizabeth's comment, "Do we have to look at another electron microscope?" Another tool of the times was the ultracentrifuge, an expensive machine that could be used with or without other physical or chemical techniques. Another experimental technique available was tissue culture – the ability to grow human cells in petri dishes in the lab. Surgically removed tissues were used to establish the cultures. Cancer cells often worked best, as they could often be immortalized to produce an endless supply. One of the best examples was the HeLa cell line from Henrietta Lacks. This became famous among biological scientists who used the cells for everything from growing viruses to testing the toxicity of cosmetics.[33] Having had my PhD training in a cancer research laboratory with ample support from the recently established Virus Cancer Program of the National Cancer Institute, I had experience with these techniques.

The late 1960s and early 1970s was also the dawn of molecular biology. The new techniques invented by biochemists over the next 15–20 years would revolutionize research in genetics and virology. Lab experiments then seemed to move into a fast-forward phase and originality in thought, hypothesis, design, and analysis seemed to be the only limitations. Technology was no longer a major restriction. No area of opportunity benefited more than drug discovery, especially for drugs that seemed hardest to develop, like those for cancer and AIDS. The new techniques allowed virologists to identify and analyze target genes by cloning and then sequencing to determine each letter in their DNA. We could even use site-specific mutagenesis and make mutations to evaluate the effect on the protein that was the product of the altered gene sequence. As DNA sequencing became easier, cancer researchers could compare the whole complement of DNA from cancer cells to the DNA of normal cells from the same organ to see what mutational problem had resulted from the error. The mutational change could then be identified and targeted at the protein level to correct the damage.

Most viruses are like animals or people in that they have a set of genes (people have about 20,000 genes whereas most viruses have 10–40 genes). The genes in people are made of a DNA code. The DNA is then transcribed to "messenger" RNA, normally with a perfect copy of the code. The RNA is then translated into proteins where each subunit is again a perfect code sequence of amino acid strands. The protein then functions as an enzyme to catalyze, digest, or assemble molecules in each cell, to send signals between cells or to build the cell structure. Viruses, lacking most of the specialized genes that cells have, can only replicate in cells, dependent on the cell machinery. When viruses replicate, they produce many progeny virus particles, which in turn usually cause cell damage. The accumulation of cell damage then becomes disease or pathology at the level of the host person. As replicating viruses get released by the damaged cells of an infected person and transmitted to someone else via body fluids, we have the start of what might become an epidemic.

Viruses are usually classified as DNA or RNA according to which type of genome is represented in their mature form of particles that get transmitted between people. The viruses of herpes, smallpox, and cervical cancer are examples of viruses classified by their DNA type, and their replication cycle is similar to that of human cells. The viruses of COVID, flu, and Ebola are examples of RNA viruses. They have no DNA stage and have their own mechanism to copy parental RNA into progeny RNA for the next generation of virus particles. Whole cells can't do that, and RNA-to-RNA copying results in many more genetic errors or mutations. This in turn causes a high degree of genetic variation, with rapid evolution of new virus strains, a situation well illustrated by COVID or flu.

HIV and the related HTLV and FeLV leukemia viruses represent an even more unusual group of viruses, called retroviruses. Retro, of course, means backward. Retroviruses like HIV are the only form of life that copies their genes backward – from RNA to DNA, rather than from DNA to RNA. Their most important gene product or protein then is the backward reverse transcriptase enzyme, a function they need that viruses can't get anywhere else in nature. Copying RNA, as both COVID viruses and retroviruses do, whether making more RNA (COVID) or new DNA (HIV), is very prone to making errors. In both cases, this leads to more mutations and more progeny virus with variations. But retroviruses have another feature that makes them unique. They surgically insert or integrate their entire genome into the chromosomal DNA of the infected human cell, which is done by another enzyme unique to these viruses called integrase. This allows them to go silent and hide until some stimulation of the cell comes along later to awaken them from latency.

So it follows that one of the first choices for targeting antiviral drugs to HIV was reverse transcriptase inhibitors like azidothymidine (AZT), which is also called zidovudine (ZDV). Quite a few other reverse transcriptase inhibitors were developed soon after.

Dr. Samuel Broder, an oncologist who was head of the National Cancer Institute, a colleague and also a friend, was the first to show that AZT, a discarded cancer drug, inhibited replication of HIV.[120] The second unique enzyme of HIV, the integrase, also turned out to be a target for another very effective class of drugs, the integrase inhibitors.

Several other classes of AIDS drugs soon followed. The anti-AIDS drugs were usually classified according to the stage of the viral life cycle they blocked, like cell entry inhibitors, reverse transcriptase inhibitors, integrase inhibitors, and protease inhibitors that interfere with assembly of progeny virus particles. Different subclasses of reverse transcriptase inhibitors were also identified. Some, like AZT or ZDV, work by binding a particular active site of the enzyme. Others, like nevirapine (NVP) or efavirenz (EFV), represent a different class of drugs because they work at a separate place on the reverse transcriptase molecule. The goal of effective therapy is to select several drugs that each have different mechanisms of action to use together.

By the early 1990s, AIDS was the leading cause of death for young men, and such drugs were desperately needed. When the first drug, AZT, was used alone in the late 1980s, it had some beneficial effect, but it usually only lasted for 6 months or less. The effect was so brief because mutant drug-resistant variants of HIV soon developed to evade the benefit of the drug. With longer use and higher doses, most drugs also had some serious side effects like gastrointestinal disturbances, anemia, or nerve toxicities. By the mid-1990s, quite a few more drugs had been developed. When used in strategic combinations, both the adverse side effects and the rapid mutational evolution to drug resistance could usually be avoided.

Another big issue that clinicians faced when drugs first became available was "when to treat." Most felt that you should not treat every person who tested positive for HIV, but wait until there were signs of clinical deterioration. The first available tests for HIV showed only whether or not the person was infected, but they didn't show whether the infection was very recent with few signs and symptoms or whether the patient had advanced disease. The cardinal indicator of advanced disease was a loss of blood lymphocytes, particularly the subset of lymphocytes called CD4 or T4, because they are the drivers of immune responses. Patients in the early stages of AIDS, like normal healthy adults, usually had more than 500 such cells per cubic centimeter of blood. End-stage AIDS patients had below 200, sometimes almost none. CD4 cell numbers could be easily monitored with a machine that used a small blood sample. Early guidelines suggested that patients should not be treated until they fell below 400 or even 300 T4 cells. This proved to be a mistake. Later guidelines indicated that patients should be treated as soon as they were detected as HIV positive, even if the T4 cells were at normal levels.

Soon after, tests were developed to determine viral load (VL) in patients' blood. This soon proved to be an accurate indicator for how well patients were doing, especially for monitoring how well the therapy was working. If the VL was 50,000 or more per cubic centimeter of blood, the patient was in serious trouble. For some patients with a million or more VL, death was imminent unless they received effective treatment very soon. Patients who were doing well on the drug regimen had VL levels below 400. With the best treatment regimens that later became available, VL might drop below detectable levels. In such cases, the infected person had so little virus replication he or she was not even infectious enough to transmit to others.

The VL test was based on a new genetic technique called polymerase chain reaction (PCR). It is based on the amplification of genetic sequences, the same tests detectives use to determine the identity of a criminal suspect based on DNA contamination. It seems ironic that the test was developed by Dr. Kary Mullis, a quirky chemist who won the Nobel Prize for his discovery, while also joining Peter Duesberg in his declarations that AIDS was not caused by HIV. Mullis was a promoter of astrology, a climate change denialist, and an advocate of psychedelic recreational drugs like LSD.

By the late 1990s or 2000, drug treatment in the United States and Europe had improved so much that patients could live an almost normal life if they took their drugs on schedule. As time went on, the drugs also proved valuable for post-exposure prophylaxis (PEP), as when a phlebotomist or lab worker might accidentally nick themselves with an HIV-containing blood sample. By the 2010s, the drugs could also be used for pre-exposure prophylaxis (PrEP) to prevent uninfected high-risk people from getting infected. By the 2020s, more than 30 HIV drugs were available, some in injectable delayed action combinations so that the patients would only need to take one dose every few months.

When first available in the late 1990s, however, the drug combinations were very expensive, perhaps \$15,000 to \$20,000 per year. The next dilemma was that the vast majority of patients were in Africa or other poor regions of the world and thus doomed to die because they couldn't afford the drugs. Political controversies ensued. Andrew Natsios, George W. Bush's head of the US Agency for International Development (USAID), embarrassed himself by declaring that Africans wouldn't take the drugs properly because they didn't have watches to tell time. A Harvard colleague, Dr. David Bangsberg, then published a series of papers showing that adherence to taking the drugs on schedule was not an impediment for their use in Africa.[121] I recall attending seminars at Harvard where many of us questioned the inequities of AIDS treatment for the developing world. My colleagues Drs. Ken Freedberg and Rochelle Walensky devoted much of their research to showing how AIDS treatment could be cost effective by saving young, productive lives, even in Africa. Rochelle would later become Joe Biden's first director of the CDC.

In 2001, Dr. Jeff Sachs, an economist colleague at Harvard's Kennedy School of Government, invited me and other faculty members to sign a letter to the US government and the Global Fund urging action to fund treatment for AIDS in the developing world. Eventually things happened, including the President's Emergency Plan for AIDS Relief (PEPFAR).

As we studied the AIDS epidemic in Africa, it became clear that the most prevalent subtypes of HIV were all different from the HIV-1B that was causing the epidemic in the United States and Europe. This raised the question of whether the drugs would work as well against the HIVs in Africa. Of particular interest was the HIV-1C of southern Africa, which was spreading faster than any of the other strains.[76] We decided we should conduct treatment trials there to assure potential donors that the drugs would work and that drug resistance could be avoided. After analyzing various drug-resistant HIVs that emerged in southern Africa, we found that they had some differences in the profile of drug-resistance mutations, but only rarely did they cause major problems.[122]

At first, the amazing progress on drug development did little to help with the HIV problem in Africa. But eventually things changed. Some help came from celebrities. I recall a small meeting in the 1990s with Mother Teresa in Rome where she called for more action in the developing world. Bono also brought attention to the problem. Magic Johnson of the Los Angeles Lakers became a symbol of drug success when he resumed playing professional basketball after a few years of effective treatment. The World Health Organization (WHO), private organizations like the Bill and Melinda Gates Foundation, and some drug companies like Merck and Bristol Myers Squibb also helped. The George W. Bush White House eventually got behind the cause to address these inequities on drug access.

The next and current challenge for HIV/AIDS is how to find a cure that will avoid the need for lifelong drug treatment. The viral genome remains as latent DNA, even in people who have been successfully treated. The current challenge is to eliminate not just free virus but also latently infected cells. This has been accomplished a couple of times but thus far only by accident. The first case was commonly known as the "German patient." He was actually an HIV-positive American student studying in Berlin when he developed leukemia along with his HIV/AIDS. The treatment protocol for the leukemia involved lethal irradiation to kill all leukemia cells, followed by bone marrow transplantation from a donor to restore the essential blood and immune cell functions needed for survival. By chance, the bone marrow donor had a rare mutation in his cells called delta 32. HIV, which has to infect cells via a cell surface receptor called CCR5, could no longer infect this patient because the transplanted cells had defective CCR5 due to the delta 32 allele. This AIDS resistance gene was discovered by a geneticist friend, Dr. Stephen O'Brien, in 1996 when he was at the National Cancer Institute.[123] He found, however, that the protective gene was only present in 1% of Caucasians and perhaps even a smaller proportion of Africans.

Using this approach would obviously not be possible as a general cure for AIDS for numerous reasons. Bone marrow transplantation itself has a higher mortality than AIDS when patients are on good chemotherapy, and finding delta 32 donors of the right transplant type would be almost impossible. Other types of gene therapy are not out of the question. As a general approach, gene therapy looked more promising some years ago. Our research group and others designed some therapeutic genes that might block HIV.[124] But vectors that would be needed to deliver the genes were not forthcoming, and the chemotherapy drugs worked much better than we anticipated. It would be fair to say that drugs have already saved the lives of tens of millions of AIDS patients.

chapter eighteen

Thailand

In the late 1980s, UNAIDS, a division of the World Health Organization, announced with great concern that the epidemic of HIV/AIDS had moved into Asia. Many thought the virus would run amok in big countries like China and India, as it did in Africa, putting most of the world's population at risk. I had several discussions on the topic with my research staff, which included doctoral students from Japan, Taiwan, and China. All thought we should get involved. I contacted a colleague at Harvard, Dr. Rapin Osathanondh, who said he could contact some of his former medical school classmates and friends back in Bangkok to help me if I went to Thailand. In fact, Rapin's father was a former president of Mahidol University, and his uncle, Anand Panyarachun, was a former Thai ambassador to the United States and a future prime minister of Thailand. Soon after, I had an invitation from Dr. Natth Bharmarapravati, then the president of Mahidol University, to come to Thailand. The Mahidol Medical School was known as the best in Thailand and one of the best in Asia.

The letter from Natth was an invitation to survey the medical faculty and senior staff of the affiliated hospitals and to make recommendations about which faculty and hospital units should be encouraged and supported to do AIDS research and teaching. I was asked to do this jointly with Dr. Donald Burke, a friend who was a colonel and head of the US Military HIV Research Program. I had never been to Thailand, but Don knew the country well.

Burke was a former Harvard medical student, and I served a term as chair of a committee to review the US Military HIV Research Program under his leadership. I gave that program a strong endorsement. Soon after, Bill Haseltine, a Harvard colleague, and I met with Senator Ted Stevens from Alaska, the powerful chair of the Senate Armed Forces and Appropriations Committees. I reported on the military AIDS program and offered my opinion that the program was doing well but that it would need more financial support to control the epidemic in the military. He asked how much money was needed. I said I didn't know, but I could make a survey and get back to him. He then offered: "The reason I need to know is the process. If it is more than $40 million for the year, I'd have to bring it to the Senate committee. But if it is for less than $40 million, I can probably write a work order to transfer the funds from someplace else." I said, "Just under $40 million should be enough for now." Soon after, the military AIDS research program got their supplement.

Burke was also involved with AFRIMS, the Armed Forces Research Institute of Medical Sciences, which was a bilateral unit formed between the US military and the Royal Thai Army. Also involved in the US military AIDS program under Burke at the time were Drs. Bob Redfield and Deborah Birx. During the Trump administration, Redfield would become head of the Centers for Disease Control and Prevention in Atlanta, and Birx would become White House Coronavirus Response Coordinator.

I soon flew to Bangkok to meet the people at Mahidol University. It was not an easy trip. I went first to Detroit, then on a long flight to Tokyo, and then another long flight to Thailand. There is an 11-hour time difference between Boston and Bangkok. This is about as bad as it gets when trying to fend off jet lag. Bangkok seemed exotic and exciting, with a population of 10 million people, great food, and very heavy traffic. I was put up in a hotel near the university as it could take 4–6 hours to go from one side of the city to the other.

Dr. Bharmarapravati's driver met us the next evening at the Polo Club for dinner. He briefed us on the schedule we'd follow for the next 2½ days. We soon learned more about the new AIDS epidemic in Thailand. After a few sporadic cases, the first real wave was in injection drug users (IDUs) in late 1987, with explosive expansion to infect about 30% of that population within a year. By 1989, there was another wave. This time it was sexual transmission, with rates of HIV infection going from about 1% to 40% in female sex workers within a single year. Thailand had a large industry of commercial sex workers. Young teenaged girls from the north of the country, especially the regions around Chiang Rai and Phayao, would move to the Bangkok region as sex workers and then return to the north after a few years. In this case, many would be returning to die. Young men in the Royal Thai Army also developed high rates of HIV infection, presumably because of their access to the female sex workers.

Soon after, we submitted our report to Natth. We mentioned that the faculty had some talented researchers but needed more equipment, lab space, and funds to get something done. I offered to help train some people at Harvard and vowed to help find some funds for training. Dr. Chantapong Wasi, a senior microbiologist, impressed us with her knowledge and cordial demeanor. She identified several young researchers who might be sent to our Boston lab within months. Two, Drs. Ruengpong Sutthent and Prasert Auewarakul, would go back to Thailand after spending 1–2 years in our lab in Boston. Soon after, they would become leaders in AIDS research in Thailand. Recognizing that HIV rates were highest in the north, we also made contact with Dr. Vicharn Vithayasai, a leading researcher at Chiang Mai University there, and he also sent us a junior colleague, Chatchawann Apichartpiyakul.

To do studies with Thai viruses, we would need blood samples from Thai patients. Both Chantapong and Vicharn shipped samples, but they were delayed in transit and then held in US Customs to be examined by officials who were overly concerned about infectious agents, especially HIV. By the time we got them, the virus in the samples was dead. Dr. Tun-Hou Lee of our group then came to the rescue. Tun-Hou is from Taiwan and a master negotiator. Tun-Hou volunteered to go to Bangkok to get the next batch of HIV samples so he could negotiate his way through customs and immigration checks at both ends. He was not only successful, but he actually arrived and immediately returned with the samples on the same plane, after the airline switched crews and departed after only a few hours on the ground in Bangkok. We got our samples, and Mary Fran McLane, our cell culture expert, grew out quite a few Thai AIDS viruses.

Soon I got another break. Deeda Blair, a friend from the Board of the Lasker Foundation, called to say that Princess Chulabhorn of the Thai Royal Family was coming to New York and that she could arrange for me to meet her. The Royal Family is revered in Thailand. The Princess received a doctorate from Mahidol University and heads the Chulabhorn Research Institute in Bangkok. Her institute does environmental and medical research, and she rapidly developed a keen interest in AIDS research. I was soon invited to a luncheon held in her honor in New York with about 30 others. As far as I could tell, most were Thai Americans and personal friends of hers or her hostess.

I was seated at the Princess's right. She told me she was interested in AIDS and wanted to encourage me to do research in Thailand. After the main meal, we were served coffee. I noticed a man crawling on the floor behind her. I was about to get up and stop him, thinking he might be a stalker. She said it was no problem as he reached up, still on his knees, to put cream in her coffee. I was embarrassingly unfamiliar with the etiquette practiced by staff when serving the Royal Family. She invited me to visit her in Bangkok, and I invited her to visit our lab in Boston.

The next time I went to Bangkok, I let her know in advance. She asked that I call her when I arrived. On that visit, I checked into the legendary Oriental Hotel, then the best hotel in Thailand and one of the best in Asia. I had a regular room, but of course it was very nice. About 2 hours after check-in and already asleep, I got a call from the front desk. The fellow said he was extremely embarrassed but that he had put me in the wrong room. I wondered whether someone else had previously checked into the same room, but I saw no evidence of that. He said the manager and the valet would come to my room immediately to help me check into a better room. They came and took me to another section of the hotel. My new

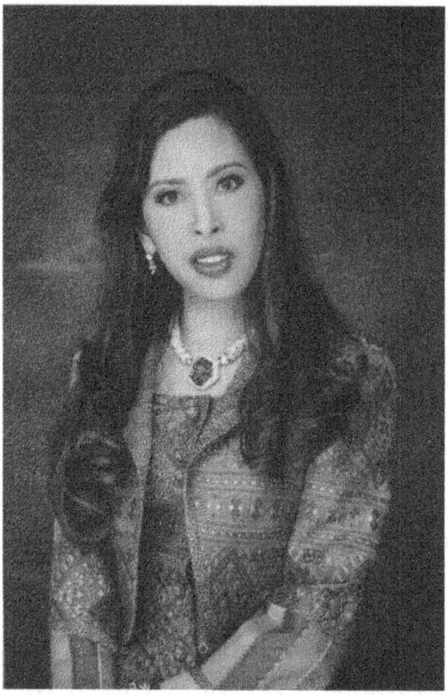

Figure 18.1: Princess Chulabhorn

"room" was an opulent four-room suite with very high ceilings and a valet on call. I said there must be some mistake – that I didn't want or need this. The manager said, "You must, it was arranged by the Royal Family and of course there is no charge to you." I was also given instructions to call a number at the royal palace, which I did the next morning.

Two days later, I was to go to the Chitralada Palace, which is where the Royal Family lives, to have tea with the Princess. She sent a car to pick me up at the Oriental. It was a large limousine with the insignia for the Royal Family on the side. As we went through the city and stopped for traffic, I saw many people dash up to the car and try to look in, but it had one-way glass on the sides so I could see out but they couldn't see me. Obviously, they thought it might be a member of the Royal Family. How disappointed they'd be if they found out it was only me. I had tea with the Princess and two colleagues, who also offered their help. The Chitralada Palace was not quite what I expected, with modern architecture rather than the tall spires of the Grand Palace, but it did have an impressive moat. Princess Chulabhorn did accept my invitation to come to Boston, and she came about a year later. She gave a talk at Harvard about AIDS in Thailand. She still sends me a Christmas card at the holiday season.

By the early 1990s, we had analyzed quite a few viruses from Thailand, both from Bangkok and from Chiang Mai, the largest city in the north. As expected, there were two distinct viruses associated with the different epidemics based on type of transmission. Patients who are injection drug users (IDUs) had HIV-1B, the same virus that causes almost all infections in the United States and Europe but was now absent in the heterosexual epidemic in Africa.[125] The heterosexual epidemic in Thailand, which accounted for 90% or more of the cases, was linked to a different virus called HIV-1E, or sometimes HIV-1A/E. This virus was from Africa, especially the region around the Central African Republic.

The quandary we had to explain was why the HIV-1B didn't seem to transmit as well as HIV-1E, or any of the other African viruses, by heterosexual contact. My hypothesis was that the HIV-1E and other African-type viruses were better able to infect cells that would be most exposed in vaginal sex, as compared to HIV-1B. We reviewed the microscopic anatomy of the sex organs. The logical target seemed to be Langerhans cells (LC). LC are present in the skin in small numbers but are especially dense in sexual mucosal tissues, particularly the junction of the vagina with the uterine cervix and on the foreskin of the penis.

We sought to grow the LC in the lab and then test the different viruses to see which would grow best in this cell type. Getting the human tissue samples was difficult as we needed fresh samples discarded from uterine surgeries. Our Thai-American friend Dr. Rapin actually did quite a few surgeries on uterine cancer patients and could give us some samples. We were also given some penile foreskin tissues that were discarded from routine male circumcisions. Drs. Luis Soto-Ramirez and Victor Peña in my group spent many hours trying to tease out and grow the cells. Eventually they were successful.

In a paper published in *Science*, we found that the Thai E viruses regularly grew better in LC than Thai or US B viruses.[126] We also tested some other African viruses from the heterosexual epidemic there. They too fit the pattern of the HIV-1E heterosexual viruses from Thailand, not the Thai or US B viruses. Other scientists did studies that enhanced the importance of our results, such as showing that chimps could be infected better vaginally with HIV-1E than with HIV-1B.[127] Our paper in *Science* received much attention. Among other invitations, I was invited to give a keynote address at the International Meeting of Langerhans Cell Researchers in Austria. Until then, I hadn't known there was such an organization.

Our research group had begun a series of meetings on HIV/AIDS in both Bangkok and Chiang Mai to better understand the epidemic in the region. We often worked jointly with the contingent from the US military as we both had interest in developing a vaccine that might be tested in Thailand. The Thai government seemed to be serious about controlling the epidemic. Mechai Viravaidya, a Thai senator, became an activist promoting AIDS education and condom use. He would sometimes dress up as a giant condom to appear at rallies of young people. Condoms were then often called "mechais" in Thailand. Under Prime Minister Anand, Rapin's uncle, the very successful "100% Condom Program" was established.[128] The program was sold particularly well in the Thai military, where a significant proportion of the men claimed they used several overlapping condoms at one time to ensure protection from HIV. Within a year or two, there was an obvious downturn in the rate of new HIV infections.

In 1992, the Harvard Medical Area had a meeting to celebrate the 100-year anniversary of Prince Mahidol, after whom the Bangkok university was named. I had nothing to do with the idea but was invited to speak at the celebration. I learned that Prince Mahidol had obtained his MD at Harvard and another degree at the School of Public Health in the 1920s. The Thai Royal Family was represented at the event by Princess Sirindhorn, the older sister of Princess Chulabhorn whom I had met earlier. When

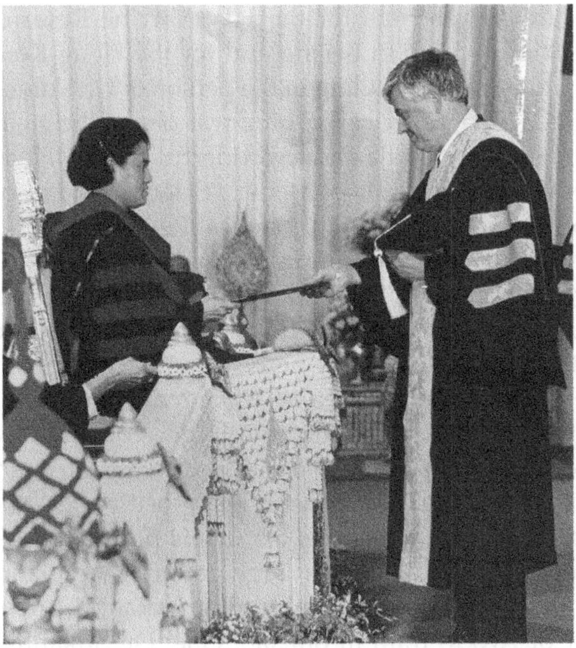

Figure 18.2: Princess Sirindhorn, Max Essex

I spoke, I expressed my sincere gratitude for welcoming me to their country.

The Thai people always seemed eager to share credit. My research there generated some useful results to help understand the epidemic, and we trained several outstanding young scientists who later did important work in the country, but it wasn't me who developed the very effective national prevention program. Nevertheless, I was given an award by Prime Minister Anand in 1999 and an honorary degree from Mahidol University in 2001. The honorary degree was presented by Princess Sirindhorn, but I was also suspicious that my friend Pornchai Matangkasombut, who was then president of the university, was somehow involved.

During the early to mid-1990s, our activities increased substantially in Asia. Along with the many trips to Thailand and Taiwan,

I was on advisory boards for the HIV Vaccine Research Center under Dr. Yiming Shao in Beijing and for the Hong Kong Cancer Institute. India was also calling in the person of Dr. Vulimiri Ramalingaswami. Rama, as we called him, was one of the great medical leaders of his time in India and a wonderful person. He was director of the All India Institute of Medical Sciences and also director-general of the Indian Council of Medical Research.

India was also experiencing a new and frightening HIV epidemic or, like Thailand, two new epidemics. The first, like Thailand, was linked to HIV-1B in IDUs. It was concentrated in the northeast, around Manipur, where the virus appeared to come from the golden triangle area of Myanmar/Burma, which had Thailand on the other side. But the larger epidemic was in the heterosexual population, where about 20% of all patients with sexually transmitted diseases were HIV positive.[129] Although the overall rate in adults was about 0.5%, this projects to 4–5 million people because India is such a large country. We planned some research with Rama, and several young Indian researchers came for a year or two to train in our lab. One, Dr. Srikanth Tripathy, analyzed representative viruses from the heterosexual epidemics in the Delhi and Mumbai regions and found that they were related to the HIV-1C from southern Africa.[130] Tripathy went back to an important position of leadership in the National AIDS Research Institute in Pune.

India is a very large country with many poor people who are usually not seen by international visitors or even the Indian government. Even blood transfusions were a serious problem in the early 1990s. Good tests were available to screen for HIV, but they were often not used to avoid the cost. It was estimated that half of the blood supply came from paid donors, many of whom were HIV positive. Most cities had a thriving sex industry, from the caged girls managed by pimps in Mumbai to the hijras of Madras – eunuchs and transsexuals who sell sex in the busy markets. One study estimated that 70% of the long-distance truckers had sexually transmitted diseases, and they averaged up to 200 sexual encounters per year.

The challenges of the HIV/AIDS epidemic in India seemed overwhelming to me, even more so than those in Thailand. Remarkably, the government made good progress, and by 2000, they were doing better than most of the countries hit by the same virus, HIV-1C, in Africa. By the late 1990s, our lab would turn much of our attention to the HIV-1C epidemic in southern Africa.

chapter nineteen

Pediatric AIDS and Princess Diana

By the early 1990s, it was apparent that HIV/AIDS was becoming a major problem in infants and children. This was especially true in those places in the world where the epidemic was primarily due to heterosexual transmission, like sub-Saharan Africa and Thailand. As more young pregnant women were infected, up to 40% of their newborn infants would also become infected. No adequate treatments were available, and most children would die by 2 or 3 years of age. In the United States and Europe, doing sterile Cesarean section surgery for delivery with HIV-positive women could reduce the proportion of infant infections, but this was not available for most situations in Africa.

In 1992, a husband-and-wife team of French physicians, Drs. Marc and Sophie Lallemant, applied to do a sabbatical leave with me in Boston. Marc was a pediatrician, and Sophie was a microbiologist. They were on leave from ORSTOM, a French government agency doing development research in the Global South, based in Brazzaville in the Republic of the Congo. In Brazzaville, they had been working with a cohort of HIV-positive pregnant women to seek factors that might be associated with maternal-infant transmission of HIV.

They found that the rate at which HIV-infected pregnant women would infect their newborn infants was 40% and that women who had more severe signs and symptoms of clinical AIDS were more likely to transmit.[131] We discussed using an antibody approach, as earlier studies of AIDS patients in our lab had shown differences in

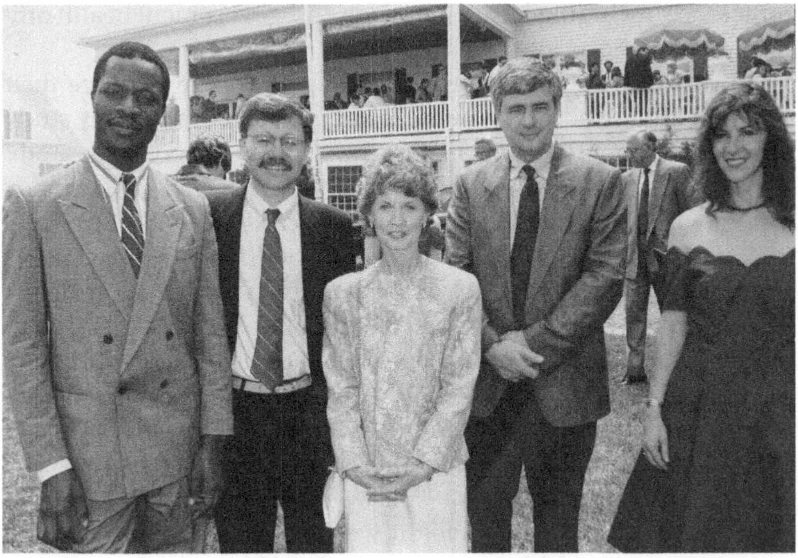

Figure 19.1: Oscar Kashala, Marc Lallemant, Elizabeth Essex, Max Essex, Sophie Lallemant

HIV antibodies that could be used as correlates for clinical staging. We then renewed a collaboration with Dr. Francis Barin, a French scientist who had earlier trained with us and was now at the University of Tours. A clear correlation was found between maternal transmission and levels of antibodies to selected pieces of the outer envelope protein of HIV, the gp120.[132]

While in our lab, the Lallemants remarked that they had difficulties accomplishing their goals in Brazzaville. I recommended that they consider moving their program to Thailand, where I had been so impressed by the cooperation from the Thai people. In particular, it seemed that northern Thailand might be appropriate because many of the Bangkok sex workers originated from there. Returning to their home region as young women, a significant fraction would be HIV positive and pregnant. I introduced Marc to my contacts in Thailand, including Dr. Vicharn Vithayasai at Chiang Mai University in the north. Together we organized an HIV/AIDS conference, including local physicians and government health officials who might be interested.

As we were making plans for Marc and Sophie to move their program to northern Thailand, results from an important study on prevention of HIV transmission from HIV-positive mothers to their infants was published in the *New England Journal of Medicine* by the pediatric AIDS clinical trials group.[133] The study trial, designated ACTG 076, was conducted in the United States and France. The goal was to see if the antiviral drug AZT could be used to prevent transmission of HIV from infected mothers to their infants. That protocol was based on the administration of AZT to the mother for the last 12 weeks before delivery and to the infant for 6 weeks after birth. The result was that this use of AZT could reduce infant infections by two-thirds as compared to the placebo with no AZT. Although this result was impressive, many international public health experts felt it was impractical for application in most countries of Africa or even Thailand because of complexity and high cost.

After consultation with Dr. Ken McIntosh, a pediatric expert on HIV at Harvard, we designed a new scheme to test AZT in a shortened, simpler way that might be easier for pregnant women to follow. The new Lallemant plan for testing in northern Thailand would compare the longer use of AZT, as in ACTG 076, to shorter courses of AZT in the mother and/or the infant. Marc submitted the new design, which had no placebo arm, as a proposal for funding to the US National Institutes of Health (NIH). The new design was an "equivalence" trial to determine whether shorter doses of AZT would work as well as the longer doses of the earlier ACTG 076 trial.

The NIH review committee rejected the application, primarily on the grounds that a placebo arm, where some mother/infant pairs received no drug, should have been included. This set off a major debate about the ethical requirements needed for conducting such trials in developing countries. The position of our research team, as well as that of the Harvard Human Subjects Committee who reviewed the application first, was that it would be unethical to include a "placebo control arm" when the ACTG 076 trial had already proven that the drug worked. The debate played out in the *New England Journal of Medicine*. While two leading medical ethicists supported our position that inclusion of a placebo control group would be unethical,[134] leaders of the NIH and the CDC defended the use of a placebo control group.[135] We responded with another piece that detailed our rationale for the no-placebo position for the same issue of the *New England Journal of Medicine*. Eventually, we won the issue, and the NIH agreed to let us conduct the trial with their financial support. Some other placebo-controlled trials funded by the NIH and CDC were stopped, and the editor of the *New England Journal of Medicine* published an editorial stating that unethical studies would not be published by that journal.[136]

Our trial in Thailand was conducted, and the results were published.[137] The conclusion was that either the longer administration of AZT to the mother or the longer administration of AZT to the infant could be shortened, but not both. We celebrated with some Singha beer and rod duan, a local delicacy of bamboo caterpillars.

In 1996, Deeda Blair, the co-chair of the Harvard AIDS Institute Advisory Board, introduced me to her close friend Marguerite Littman. Marguerite had initiated the first major charity for AIDS in the United Kingdom when she solicited funds for the cause from hundreds of her friends. Marguerite was quite a character in her own right, counting Truman Capote, David Hockney, Elton John, and Gore Vidal among her friends. She was originally from Louisiana. After college, she moved to Hollywood to work as a voice coach. She worked with actors like Elizabeth Taylor and Paul Newman, teaching them to "speak southern" for movies like *Cat on a Hot Tin Roof*. The character Holly Golightly in *Breakfast at Tiffany's* was said to be based on Marguerite. She married Mark Littman, a British barrister, and then lived at Chester Square in London in a townhouse that was next door to the home of Margaret Thatcher. Marguerite donated both time and financial resources to our AIDS research program.

In the late 1990s, I often traveled through London to Africa for our research program in Botswana. Marguerite enjoyed entertaining and frequently offered to host a lunch or reception to raise funds at her home if I could stop by on my way to Africa. I often

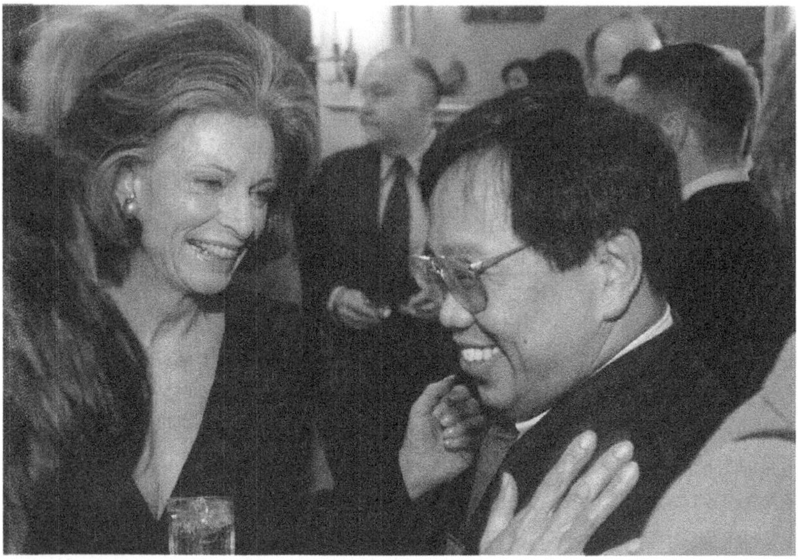

Figure 19.2: Deeda Blair, Tun-Hou Lee

did. Her husband, Mark, was a barrister who was also a Queen's Counsel, and Marguerite was a close friend of Diana, Princess of Wales. Working with Deeda Blair, she received a gift of Diana's dresses to be auctioned at Christie's in New York with the Harvard AIDS Institute (HAI) to be listed as a recipient of the proceeds.

In the spring of 1997, the Advisory Board of the HAI voted for Princess Diana to be the recipient of the annual award for AIDS advocacy. The award was usually presented at a dinner in Boston or New York. I sent a letter to Princess Diana mentioning that she was selected as a recipient of the award and asking whether she could attend a dinner in New York for the presentation. The Princess soon replied with a counterproposal. She said she felt honored and was grateful for the award but felt that a dinner in New York would focus too much attention on her and not enough on the needs related to AIDS issues in the developing world. For about 6 months, I exchanged correspondence and phone calls with the Princess and her senior staff, Michael Gibbins and Angela

Hordern. After I described our activities in Africa and Asia, Diana mentioned that she'd like to accompany me on a visit to one of our research sites. As Michael Gibbins explained to me, "If the Princess only attends a dinner in New York, too much attention will be on the wrong things, like what she is wearing and which government officials and society leaders were included."

The Princess then invited me to meet with her for tea at Kensington Palace, a residence for the British Royal Family in London. We met for about an hour on the afternoon of June 9, 1997. I gave more detail about our research and training programs. She described the trip she took to Angola the year before for the International Red Cross. The purpose of that trip was to emphasize the need to remove landmines in countries formerly at war to prevent injuries and deaths in innocent children. After 10 or 15 minutes, she released her aide, Michael Gibbins, saying we could work out the details. After discussing our programs in Africa and Thailand, it was clear that she favored Thailand because it would allow her to emphasize the importance of HIV/AIDS in pregnant women and infants. I mentioned that our mother/infant programs were in the north of Thailand, especially in rural areas near Chiang Mai and Chiang Rai. I also mentioned that I knew Princess Chulabhorn in Thailand and that she would probably be happy to help with the program as she was particularly interested in AIDS research. Diana countered that she would love to go to the north but would prefer to avoid any formal activities in Bangkok or with the Thai Royal Family, believing that it might distract the press so they would pay less attention to the issues of AIDS. We agreed to travel to Thailand. With my approval, her office then released a press statement: "Diana, Princess of Wales, will visit Thailand from 22–26 November 1997. She will be accompanied by the chairman and certain of the trustees of the Harvard AIDS Institute and will visit some of the facilities and research programs developed by the Institute in Thailand."

When my time was up for the meeting with Diana, an aide came into the parlor to say that my car was waiting and that she would escort me out. Diana dismissed the aide and insisted on walking me to the car. She stood by the taxi and waved as I left. The driver was thrilled and said, "Wow, you must be important" as we drove away.

Back in Boston, we made preparations for the Thailand trip. My wife Elizabeth and I were to accompany the Princess along with Maurice Tempelsman and Deeda Blair, the co-chairs of the Institute's Advisory Council, and Dr. Ric Marlink, our executive director. Dr. Rapin Osathanondh, my Thai friend at Harvard, had helped tremendously with the arrangements. His uncle, former prime minister Anand Panyarachun, who was also brought in to the government to calm the coup in 1992, would meet us in Thailand. The Siam Commercial Bank would provide us with a plane to fly from Bangkok to Chiang Mai, where we would be met by Marc and Sophie Lallemant. Countess Albina du Boisrouvray from Switzerland would also fly in from Paris to meet us. Albina was also a friend. She founded the FXB Center for Health and Human Rights at Harvard and also the building that housed our research laboratories. Even more relevant in this context, Albina endowed several orphanages for children with HIV/AIDS in the Chiang Mai region.

On August 30, 1997, Elizabeth was watching the news when a bulletin surfaced about Princess Diana. My wife called me to come over as we both heard about a serious car crash in a Paris tunnel. Soon we learned that Diana was dead. Albina and others called to commiserate.

Now the hour I spent with Diana seems like a treasure. I'll always remember the little things. Her brisk walk into the parlor to greet me with a big smile, the eager way she shook my hand. During our time together, she asked many astute questions and said all the right things. It was easy to forget she was a princess. She seemed to be my – and everyone else's – friend.

The glass sculpture appreciation award we had engraved to give to Diana still sits on my office bookcase, never presented. In her parlor at Kensington Palace, I noticed many photos. All but one or two were of Prince William and Prince Harry. The only other photo I recall, situated prominently, was of Mother Theresa. It didn't look out of place.

chapter twenty

The Harvard AIDS Institute

In 1979, Dean Howard Hiatt said he wanted to recommend me for a permanent position as full professor with tenure. He said he had only one condition, which was that I also agree to serve as a department chair. When I first accepted a junior faculty position in 1972, my plan was to avoid a position that would lead to major administrative responsibilities, at least for the next 15–20 years. Chairs of some departments told me they spent half or more of their time on administration. It seemed logical that the most important responsibility of the chair would be to recruit the best junior faculty. "If new faculty are really good, they'll just want to be left alone," I was told by one department chair I respected. It turned out he was right. At Harvard, in lab departments such as ours, new faculty recruits who don't work out soon leave. The school provides little to support research beyond a starter package for new faculty. Without outside research funding, one cannot hire lab techs, buy equipment, or pay for research supplies. And graduate students who want to finish a PhD in a reasonable time period logically stay away from faculty advisors who don't have a robust lab to pay for their research expenses. Faculty who have the most success getting research grants, especially government grants that also provide overhead funds, get the largest space allocations. Getting research grants is related to a scientist's ability to present new hypotheses in a believable proposal. So there is some truth to the statement that success in academic research is dependent on one's ability to raise money as the major determinant of the "up or out philosophy."

Recruitment of junior faculty is done in several ways. One is by advertising in specialty journals, such as journals in the fields of virology, microbiology, and immunology. Another is by contacting senior colleagues who are in the appropriate disciplines. In the 1980s, I knew we had to recruit an immunologist, so I contacted Dr. Baruj Benacerraf. Baruj had won the Nobel Prize in Physiology and Medicine in 1980 for his work in immunology. He was also chair of the Department of Pathology at the Harvard Medical School. He said he'd come right over to my office to talk. This seemed odd as I knew him as an old-school, traditional, and formal type of guy, many years my senior. He said he could recommend Laurie Glimcher, who was a very good immunologist. He then added, "But I don't know if you want her, because she's a woman." I told him that was even better, that we gave special credit to women and minority applicants. We hired Laurie. It was soon clear that she was a star. She got early promotion to professor, then became president of the American Association of Immunologists, and is now president of the Dana-Farber Cancer Center. I still call her if I need advice about medical expertise in rheumatology or oncology.

When rebuilding the department, I felt that we also needed expertise in tuberculosis (TB). It was clear that three infectious diseases stood in the way of development for most countries in the Global South. The three were HIV/AIDS, malaria, and TB. We already had HIV/AIDS covered and a leading malaria expert in Dr. Dyann Wirth. We'd have to find someone to develop a program on TB. I called Dr. John Mekalanos, who was probably the leading expert on disease-causing bacteria at Harvard. I knew John well, as we were both on the Scientific Advisory Board for a local biotech company, Virus Research Institute. He recommended Eric Rubin, an MD/PhD infectious disease expert interested in TB. Eric was also very successful. Our department soon became a leader in TB research. Eric is now editor-in-chief of the *New England Journal of Medicine*, one of the most prestigious positions in academic medicine.

By the late 1980s, the numbers of HIV infections were increasing very fast in US cities and in Europe but also in the rest of the world, especially Africa. Dr. Harvey Fineberg, our dean, came up with a new idea. Harvey had seen Harvard from several viewpoints. He was an undergraduate at Harvard College. Then he earned an MD degree at Harvard Medical School. That was followed by a master's in public policy from the Harvard Kennedy School, and finally a PhD from the Graduate School of Arts and Sciences. He came to me with an idea that there should be a new organizational structure, the Harvard AIDS Institute (HAI). The HAI would have representation from all parts of the university, with me in charge. It sounded intimidating, but Harvey said he had raised the idea with Derek Bok, the president of Harvard, and Derek was on board. The goal would be to get more faculty involved with the AIDS problem, especially some in disciplines not already represented, and to work together to raise funds for AIDS-related teaching and research.

By this time, I wasn't quite as intimidated by administration, having survived almost two 5-year terms as a department chair, but I still wanted to spend most of my time on teaching and research. I also knew I didn't have the glad-handing personality needed to raise funds from private donors, even if it were done with the blessing of the Harvard brass. On the other hand, the situation with AIDS certainly needed big ideas, big investment, and new approaches, and a few other universities were setting up their own AIDS research centers or institutes. So I decided to give it a try.

We already had a core group of faculty scientists who were actively collaborating on the virology, immunology, and epidemiology of AIDS, including Dr. Martin Hirsch at Massachusetts General Hospital, Dr. Bill Haseltine at the Dana-Farber Cancer Center, Dr. Jerome Groopman at the Beth Israel Deaconess Hospital, and me. A feature about our collaboration had been published in the *New York Times Sunday Magazine* in 1986.[138] With the new sanction from President Bok, who was listed as Policy Board chair, new Policy Board members were added, including Deans Daniel Tosteson and James Adelstein from the Medical School, Deans Fineberg and Blout from the School of Public Health, Dean Al Carnesale of the Kennedy School, Dean Ron Theimann of the Divinity School, Dr. Sarah Lawrence-Lightfoot of the Graduate School of Education, and Larry Tribe of the Law School. Two close friends

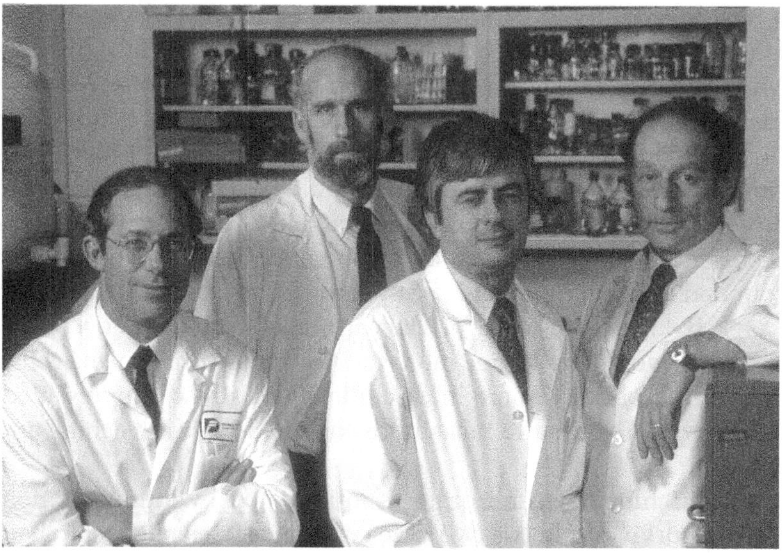

Figure 20.1: William Haseltine, Jerome Groopman, Max Essex, Martin Hirsch

and supporters of mine on the outside, Deeda Blair and Maurice Tempelsman, were also recruited as co-chairs of an International Advisory Council. With a group like this, how could we fail?

So we were thinking big. At Harvard, this usually means a new building or endowing a school as a "naming opportunity." A good example is the T.H. Chan School of Public Health, which came about when Dr. Gerald Chan and his brother Ronnie gave a gift of $360 million to the school to memorialize their father. Gerald was a doctoral student in our department and I knew him, but that probably had little or nothing to do with how he made his money, and I had nothing to do with soliciting his gift.

For HAI, the most obvious approach in thinking big was a building. Most of the Harvard AIDS researchers needed more lab space and would be happy to be housed together. The deans might also be happy if it would open up existing space that they could then use for other purposes. Our first prospect was David Geffen in Los Angeles. Geffen got rich in the recording and film

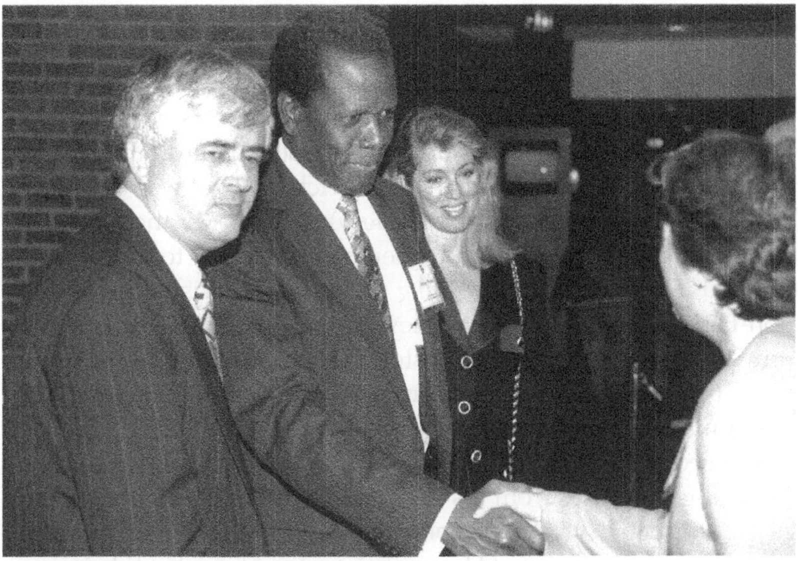

Figure 20.2: Max Essex, Sidney Poitier, Joanna Shimkus
Photo by Richard Chase.

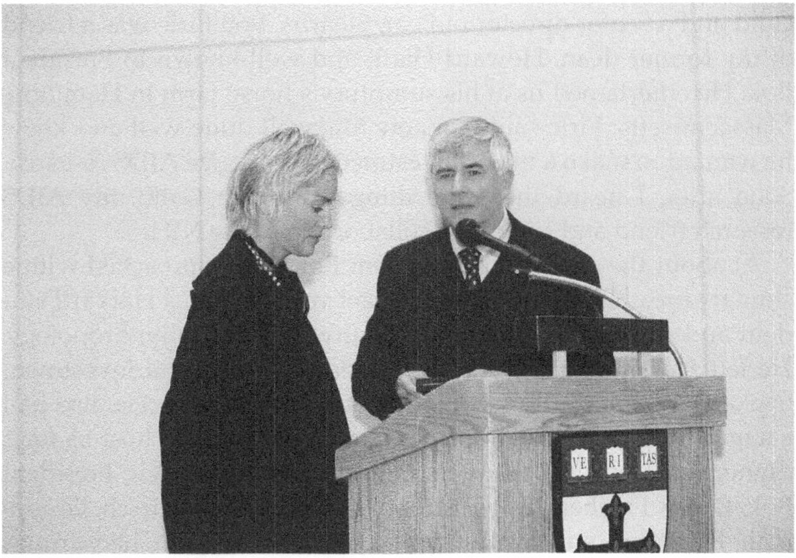

Figure 20.3: Sharon Stone, Max Essex

industries in the 1980s. He had no particular association with Harvard, but he was interested in the AIDS problem, and we had quite a few good contacts in LA. Hollywood was being decimated by AIDS, and the Harvard Club in LA was interested in helping. John Lithgow (AB '67) was on our Advisory Board, and he gave me advice for quite a few years. Ed Zwick (AB '74) was doing well in the late 1980s with both film (*Glory*) and TV. My then teenaged daughter, Carrie, was thrilled when he invited her to the set of the popular TV show *thirtysomething* on one of our visits. Some other non-Harvard notables like Sidney Poitier, Richard Gere, and Sharon Stone also made trips to Boston to help. In 1989, four of us representing HAI – Deans Fineberg and Tosteson, along with Jerry Groopman and myself – made a visit to David Geffen. We were all impressed with his beachside home in Malibu. We could even watch frolicking porpoises from his living room, which I came to think of as the ultimate Hollywood experience. But in the end, Geffen wasn't up to buying a building at Harvard. Sometime later, he did give several hundred million to rename the medical school at UCLA.

Our next prospect was Robert Maxwell. He was first suggested to us by Robert Pirie, a Harvard man, who was CEO of Rothschild and a senior director of Bear, Stearns. Bob Pirie was a friend of my former dean, Howard Hiatt, and well-known to President Bok. He entertained us at his sumptuous horse farm in Hamilton, Massachusetts. Pirie said he knew Maxwell quite well and knew he wanted to make a major investment to energize AIDS research. Soon after, I heard the same thing from Bob Gallo, my AIDS research friend and sometime collaborator at the NIH.

At about the same time, President Bok was approached with a similar story. His contact was Michael von Clemm, a Harvard student and subsequently a junior faculty member in anthropology. He left Harvard to become an immensely successful investment banker with Credit Suisse, First Boston, and others. He also had a sumptuous estate near Boston. Von Clemm was to host us for a dinner session at his home in Wellesley with Maxwell. President Bok, Deans Fineberg and Tosteson, as well as Drs. Hirsch, Groopman, Haseltine, and I would all be there. We arrived, had drinks, and Von Clemm told us that Maxwell was expected soon. He had his own helicopter, which would land on Von Clemm's heliport. The weather wasn't so good. About an hour later, Von Clemm told us that Maxwell, a Brit, would try to reschedule next time he was in New York. There never was a next time as Maxwell died soon after.

Being a spectator to some of these adventures was interesting, but it wasn't helping us do research. We needed to hire an executive director and a small staff for HAI to bring together interested faculty and students, to organize think tanks and workshops, to train students and fellows in AIDS research, and to publish updates for all interested parties. And we needed to find the financial resources to do these things.

When the HAI began, the deans of Public Health and Medicine, as well as President Bok, each contributed $50,000–$100,000 per year from their budgets for the first 3 or 4 years. At the outset, we had one other source of funds – royalties from the gp120 patent. The patent had been filed a few years before by the Harvard Patent Office with Tun-Hou Lee and me as inventors. Gp120 is the HIV molecule that is necessary for the diagnostic tests used both for AIDS disease diagnosis and for screening blood used for transfusions. The patent was issued in 1988, just about the time HAI was getting started. A dozen or more pharmaceutical and biotech companies purchased licenses from Harvard to use the gp120 technology. This was an immediate source of some modest income that would presumably go up after the companies actually made diagnostics and paid royalties on the products.

Under Harvard's usual procedures, the largest fractions of patent income would be distributed to the president's office, the dean's office, the academic department where the research was done (which was our department), and the lab where the work was done (again, our lab). In this case, the president, the dean, and I negotiated an arrangement whereby all these fractions would go to the HAI, at least for the first 2 to 3 years.

As the gp120 technology was commercialized, it soon became apparent that the licensee who appeared to have the largest market share, Abbott, was not paying royalties. Tun-Hou and I raised this with several administrators, who stated that there was little we could do. The implication was that they didn't want to be exposed to the unseemly press that might be associated with suits for patent infringement. We countered with our knowledge that the scientific argument was solid and that MIT, who had more experience with patents, had been much more aggressive about enforcement. Within about a year, a new person was appointed as head of the Harvard Office of the General Counsel. She was Margaret Marshall from Choate Hall & Stewart LLP. We learned that Ms. Marshall had a background that included patents and litigation.

We met with Ms. Marshall, or Margie, as she preferred to be called. We were very impressed. Margie was born and raised in South Africa. After a brief career protesting apartheid, she emigrated to the United States. After earning her JD from Yale Law School, she became a US citizen. We explained our situation with the gp120 patent and Harvard's reluctance to go after Abbott. She said she was on board and would handle the case herself. We were told to prepare for a court appearance. It took a while, but just as we were preparing for the court case, Margie called to say that Abbott had just settled for a $6 million payout. She had a celebration party for Tun-Hou and me, even inviting some of those who had been reluctant to challenge Abbott.

A few years later, Margie left Harvard when Governor Weld appointed her to the Massachusetts Superior Court. After a few more years, Governor Cellucci appointed her as the Chief Justice. In 2003, she wrote the majority decision for the landmark case of *Goodridge v. Department of Public Health*. This was the first case where any state found that same-sex couples have the right to marry. Some years later, even the US Supreme Court would agree. Harvard also then gave Margie an honorary doctorate. No one cheered more than Tun-Hou and I.

chapter twenty-one

Educating Scientists

HAI was just beginning about 5–10 years after the start of the AIDS epidemic. It was already clear that we were faced with a pandemic that seemed certain to last for decades and to get worse before it got better. Most researchers and professors with appropriate expertise gave lectures to anyone who would listen and in-depth detail for those who wanted more. One of my most satisfying experiences was a course on AIDS in Africa that I did for Harvard freshmen. Most of them were brilliant. I expected that. What I didn't quite expect was how appreciative, generous, and adventurous they'd be. I was so impressed that we established a semester abroad program so undergraduates could take other classes on site while participating in AIDS projects in southern Africa. They, and I, also had major interactions with African students interested in an in-depth education on HIV/AIDS. Unbeknownst to me at the time, but then to my great delight, some Harvard donors established a fellowship endowment in my name that would be used to support African students at Harvard.

A major need was to provide expertise rapidly on HIV/AIDS for developing countries in Africa and Asia. Clearly, we weren't the only ones to recognize this need. In 1988, the Fogarty International Center of the NIH established a new fund for applicants to file competing applications for the training of AIDS scientists from developing countries. A major condition was that the trainees would be required to return to their home countries following the completion of their training period. Additionally, the US host training institution who applied for the funding would be required to prove that they had adequate contacts in the developing countries to assist graduates of the program in finding jobs upon their return. We filed one of the first applications to partner with Mexico, China, Thailand, Tanzania, Taiwan, Senegal, and the Democratic Republic of Congo. Our efforts were soon rewarded with a 5-year grant for several million dollars. Soon we were required to delete China from our list because of the human rights violations around the Tiananmen Square protests, and later Taiwan because their economy grew so much they ceased to be a "developing country." But we also added Nigeria, Kenya, and Botswana. The trainees could be based at any of the Harvard schools or affiliated teaching hospitals as long as their research training was related to HIV/AIDS.

The NIH Fogarty grant would be successfully renewed every 5 years for about 30 years. It also provided seed funds for small AIDS-related research conferences, and we held these events in a wide range of places from Lubumbashi, in the Democratic Republic of Congo, and Chiang Mai, Thailand, to Boston. Among them was a series of think tanks to strategize about how to make a vaccine that included various vaccine experts like Dr. Deborah Birx. At that time, Debi was head of the US Military HIV Research Program. Later, she would go on to be an unappreciated COVID expert in the Trump White House.[139] We held regular conferences for updates on AIDS information in Senegal and Thailand, and a few in the Democratic Republic of Congo, Nigeria, Tanzania, and later Botswana. We also published two volumes of information on AIDS in Africa[79,140] and one on AIDS in Asia[141] for health-care personnel in those regions and co-edited with Dr. Vince De Vita, Tony Fauci, and others a textbook on AIDS medicine for health-care personnel in the United States and Europe.[142] The HAI also published regular updates on research topics in the *Harvard AIDS Review*.

After a relatively disappointing period on drug research progress up to the early 1990s, Dr. Richard Marlink collaborated with Dr. David Pauza at the University of Wisconsin and Martin Delaney of Project Inform to stimulate action on development of drugs for AIDS. They brought together leaders from government like Drs. Tony Fauci, Bob Gallo, and Sam Broder of the National Institutes of Health and Dr. David Kessler of the Food and

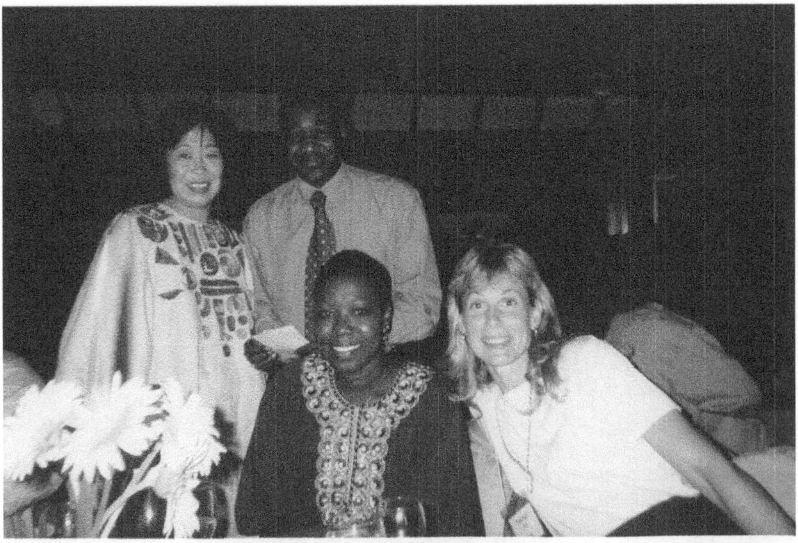

Figure 21.1: Phyllis Kanki, Souleymane Mboup, Aissatou Gueye, Debi Birx

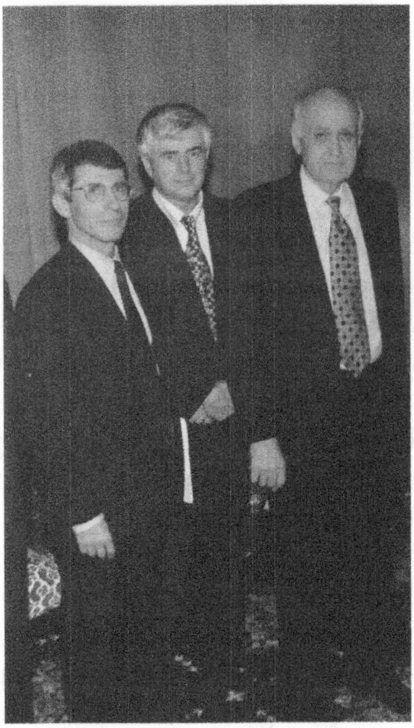

Figure 21.2: Tony Fauci, Max Essex, Maurice Hilleman

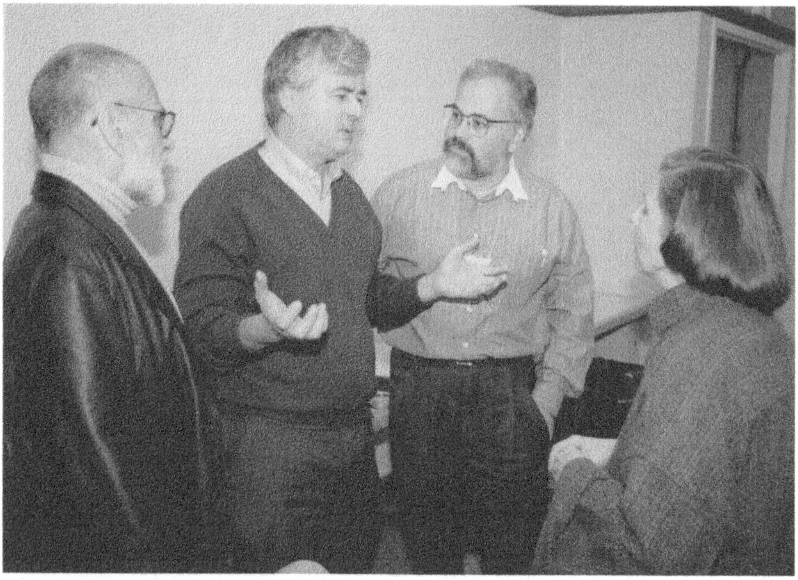

Figure 21.3: Larry Kramer, Max Essex, George Pavlakis

Drug Administration with pharmaceutical industry leaders like Dr. Maurice Hilleman of Merck, Dr. David Barry of Burroughs Wellcome, and Dr. Stephen Carter of Bristol Myers Squibb. Academics like Dr. Howard Temin from the University of Wisconsin, Dr. June Osborn from the University of Michigan, Dr. Tom Coates from the University of California at San Francisco, and our own group at Harvard were also involved. But perhaps of greatest importance, Ric Marlink sought to include substantial input from the US community of patients and activists. They included David Barr of the Gay Men's Health Crisis Center, Gregg Gonsalves and Mark Harrington of the Treatment Action Group, and perhaps most important of all, Larry Kramer.

Kramer was a playwright and film producer who co-founded the Gay Men's Health Crisis Center, which grew to be the world's largest private organization assisting people with AIDS. I got to observe Kramer's impact up close when a group of about 40 protesters started demonstrating loudly outside our conference room in Madison, Wisconsin. Larry said, "I'll handle it" and invited me to go out with him to talk to the protesters. Some recognized him and quieted the others while Larry gave a short introduction. The group immediately broke into resounding applause.

Ric Marlink also organized sessions in Boston to give updates on AIDS to leaders in the US Black community with help from Harvard faculty like Dr. Henry Louis "Skip" Gates Jr., who was head of the Department of African and African American Studies, and Drs. Cornell West and Anthony Appiah, who were then at Harvard. Ric then organized a major think tank session called Africa Now to bring together African and American leaders to organize a plan for prevention and treatment of AIDS in Africa, with several African heads of state in attendance.

Another annual activity of the HAI, usually occurring around World AIDS Day, December 1, was a series of research updates and the presentation of awards to those who had done great things to promote the cause of AIDS. One early recipient was Cleve Jones. In the early 1980s, he started the AIDS Memorial Quilt project to memorialize people who had died of AIDS. By the 1990s, it was large enough to cover the National Mall. It would later grow to exceed 50 tons.

Through these awards, we also got to know Arthur Ashe, the great tennis pro, who died of AIDS in 1993 at age 49, just a week or two after finishing his book *Days of Grace*.[143] It was believed that he became infected through a contaminated blood transfusion during bypass surgery. He spoke at the UN General Assembly and at many other places about the need to mobilize AIDS prevention. In 1992, en route to an AIDS education session with sports journalists, he stopped for a visit at my home. He was not doing well. I remember how difficult it was to control my emotions as he spoke by phone with his young daughter, Camera. Soon after, in 1993, I brought my own daughter Holly to attend a private memorial service for Arthur in Richmond, where he was born and raised. We were both deeply moved, reflecting on the blessings we had with each other and with the rest of our family.

Public education during the first decade of AIDS was mainly focused on the United States and Western Europe. By the early

1990s, African programs were getting underway. Colleagues at Johns Hopkins University established an important partnership in Uganda. Our HAI team began with a program in Senegal led by Dr. Souleymane Mboup. With Souleymane in Dakar and Phyllis Kanki in Boston, we trained a large number of AIDS experts. Le Dantec Hospital at the University Cheikh Anta Diop in Dakar, where Mboup has his lab, also served as a regional training center for UNAIDS and for other francophone West African countries, attracting students from countries like Guinea, Côte d'Ivoire, Cameroon, and Burkina Faso. Some of the students who did well and wanted more were then invited for a stint in Boston. If they did well with that, some would be accepted for a degree program.

The UNAIDS, other international agencies, and some pharmaceutical companies also invited us to teach in countries that might not have much AIDS expertise. I once spent 4 days in Niger, a very poor country that had recently experienced a military coup d'état. I was flown in on a pharmaceutical company plane, a Learjet, from France. On the way back to Paris, we stopped for fuel at an isolated concrete strip in the middle of the Sahara Desert in Algeria. Two Arab men appeared from over a hill, pulling a wagon with a large tank of fuel. After long negotiations with one of the pilots, the men pumped fuel into the plane, but only after the pilot gave them a stack of *Playboy* magazines along with the cash payment. Upon arrival in Paris, a limousine met the plane at the small Le Bourget airport. I was driven to my hotel without anyone checking my passport upon entry into the country, again emphasizing the benefits of being rich.

For teachers, perhaps the greatest reward is the accomplishments of their students. The success of mentees seems even more special when they have come from a modest beginning. Harvard is an ideal place for a professor to bask in the success of his students. Thumbi Ndung'u was such a student. He came from an agrarian background in rural Kenya. Along with 10 siblings, he picked coffee beans and milked the family cow. He scored unusually high in his classes, especially in math and the sciences, at the University of Nairobi. Through an opportunity from the US Agency for International Development, he had a chance to visit Harvard for a brief period of training. It was his first time out of Kenya. He so impressed his faculty adviser that he was urged to apply for a PhD program. He was accepted and chose me to be his thesis mentor. For his thesis topic, we decided that he would concentrate on HIV-1C, which is the most prevalent HIV in the world, more common than all other subtypes of HIV combined. HIV-1C has been particularly devastating in the countries of southern Africa like Botswana and the Republic of South Africa.

Thumbi started to make major research contributions while conducting his thesis research, making the first infectious clone of HIV-1C.[144] He then went on to make a hybrid virus between HIV-1C and a simian immunodeficiency virus. Taken in combination, these results allowed further research for HIV drugs and vaccines to be confident that the interventions would work against the most prevalent virus in Africa. At his graduation, Thumbi won the prize for the best doctoral thesis in the biomedical sciences for the Harvard School of Public Health.

A major problem for much of the Global South is the "brain drain." Many of the top foreign students who graduate from the best universities in the United States are unable to resist the job offers they get to stay in the United States. Along with the much higher salaries and living conditions, graduates accustomed to using advanced technologies with expensive equipment might feel they could not be successful doing the same work in Africa. The Fogarty training stipends are designed for scholars who will return to their home countries to build intellectual capacity around HIV/AIDS. After Thumbi completed his degree, he went back to Africa, initially working at the Botswana Harvard lab in Gaborone. After a few years, he moved on to a leadership position at the University of KwaZulu-Natal in South Africa. He soon received a Howard Hughes Early Career Scientist Award for his research. After a few more years, he'd receive more awards, including the KT Jeang Retrovirology Prize and a Harvard Alumni Award. Of greatest importance, he is now mentoring a large number of African PhD students in his own lab near Durban.

One of the successors to Thumbi as head of the Botswana lab was Sikhulile Moyo, who was also a Fogarty trainee with our group at Harvard. Sikhulile was from Zimbabwe, a country in turmoil and economic depression under the dictatorship of Robert Mugabe. Sikhulile was very bright, and he worked very hard, thinking he could make a difference and ameliorate the effects of viral epidemics in Africa. He made a difference for Africa and the world as the discoverer of the Omicron variant of COVID. For this, he was featured in *Time* as one of the 100 Most Influential People in 2022. This led to other awards and a decision by the World Health Organization to purchase some modern equipment to be placed in the Botswana lab for his use.

Because of the Fogarty program, hundreds of Africans became well trained to fight the AIDS epidemic on that continent. Because of their education and intelligence, most of them are also qualified to tackle new epidemics, as Sikhulile did with COVID. The recognition that many such trainees are in place to staff positions in the Global South should make us all feel a little safer when the next pandemic emerges.

chapter twenty-two

The Boston Conference

In 1988, Dr. Yamil Kouri came to my office with an idea. He thought that Harvard should file a proposal to host the 1992 meeting of the International AIDS Society in Boston. The International AIDS Conference was held every year, usually in June or July. The first conference was held in Atlanta in 1985, organized by the Centers for Disease Control and Prevention (CDC). The subsequent meetings seemed to alternate between sites in Europe and the United States, with the US meetings usually drawing in excess of 10,000 delegates. The sites for the 1990 and 1991 meetings had already been selected as San Francisco and Florence, Italy.

Kouri said he had raised the idea with Harvey Fineberg, our dean. Fineberg was supportive, according to Kouri, but they both felt it would only work if the proposal were submitted by an internationally recognized AIDS researcher such as me. I mentioned that there were several other well-known AIDS researchers at Harvard, such as Drs. Marty Hirsch, Bill Haseltine, and Jerry Groopman. All were friends and research collaborators. It was then pointed out that they wouldn't be eligible because they weren't actually based at Harvard. Although they had Harvard teaching rights and responsibilities through the Harvard Medical School, their financial and contractual arrangements were at the Harvard-affiliated hospitals, not the university itself. As we all believed the university would be much more likely than any of the hospitals to advance the money needed to organize the conference, it came back to me to be officially proposed as conference chair with Yamil as vice chair.

I first met Dr. Kouri when he invited me to be on his doctoral thesis committee. His primary advisor was a health economist in the Department of Health Policy and Management. His thesis topic was on the design of a plan to provide care for AIDS patients in San Juan, Puerto Rico, where he had most recently lived with his family. I had no expertise in economics or health policy, but he needed someone on the committee with knowledge about HIV/AIDS, so I agreed. I knew that Kouri was from Cuba, but that was about all I knew about him, except that he had recently completed a master's degree at the school. Another faculty member from his committee filled me in and suggested I read an article about Kouri from the *New York Times*.[145]

It turned out that Yamil Kouri had been a featured speaker at Harvard's last commencement ceremony in Cambridge, when he had received his master's degree. His talk, and his life, were indeed extraordinary. His speech was the highlight of the graduation ceremony for an audience of 25,000.

Kouri had been a student at Harvard College in the 1950s. He left in 1958 before completing his undergraduate degree to join Fidel Castro's revolutionary army in Cuba. By 1959, the revolution was successful. Yamil stayed in Cuba to complete medical school at the University of Havana and raise a family. He soon became the director of Cuba's National Center for Scientific Research. In a few years, he noticed that the freedom they had fought for was rapidly diminishing and the government was turning into a dictatorship. He and some other young idealists began to voice concern to the new Castro government. Kouri was then sentenced to prison. The first 2½ years were in solitary confinement without light, clothing, or books. He was then released from solitary confinement but still imprisoned for another 12 years with other political dissidents. While there, he provided medical advice to the other prisoners, limited by his lack of access to medical instruments and drugs.

In 1979, Kouri was released from Cuba with the first group of political prisoners set free by Castro as part of a negotiated agreement with President Jimmy Carter. Two Jesuit priests from Puerto Rico went to Cuba to receive Kouri and others, and he went to San

Juan, where he was reunited with his family. In 1987, I was invited to be commencement speaker at Columbia's Medical School. I assumed they invited me because they wanted to hear about HIV/AIDS. I spoke some about AIDS but even more about the Kouri saga, which had impressed me, and the lessons we should all be learning from his experience.

In 1988, I was invited to Cuba to view and comment on their policy on HIV/AIDS. The rumors were that the government was testing the entire population for HIV and locking up those who were HIV positive. It was a strange trip. Howard Hiatt, an MD policy expert, went with me. At that time, the only readily available route was to go from Canada. We were told that a small chartered plane could also take us from Miami, but it wasn't officially sanctioned. We left Miami at 2 am, when the airport appeared to be closed. After arrival in Havana, we were assigned an official escort, housed in government accommodations, and each given a large bottle of rum. We then spent 3 days meeting with the Minister of Health and his staff, and visiting numerous health-related establishments. They included primary-care facilities, hospitals for specialists, and research institutes. It was clear that the health-care sector received a large fraction of the tax income and that the government was proud of this. The research institute that the government seemed most eager to profile was the Pedro Kouri Institute of Tropical Medicine. The photo of Pedro Kouri displayed at the entrance, adjacent to a photo of Fidel Castro, revealed a remarkable resemblance to the Yamil Kouri I knew. I later learned that Pedro was Yamil's uncle.

The HIV testing was being done properly, as far as I could tell. I was unable to determine whether HIV-positive people were being locked up. One vivid memory I had was when I was leaving the country, walking out to board the small plane. My government escort pulled me aside and said, "Please, can you find a way for me to get out of Cuba?" as he handed me a handwritten card with his phone number. Later, I would hear a similar story from a few Cuban physicians who had been sent to Africa to assist with the AIDS epidemic. They wanted to know if Botswana or another African country would give them political asylum.

The Harvard AIDS Institute (HAI) was an appropriate organization for filing our application to host the 1992 international AIDS meeting in Boston. Along with the several hundred thousand dollars allocated to HAI by the deans and the president's office, the central administration approved an advance of several million dollars that we could use to hire the people and acquire the services needed to prepare for the meeting. This would, however, be a loan, to be paid back from funds collected from the corporate entities who would purchase space for commercial display booths and from delegate registration fees. Organizations such as the World Health Organization (WHO), the US NIH, and the US CDC also had a history of contributing funds for the conference in previous years, and we would go back to them for the meeting planned for Boston. We'd also need to reserve the Boston Hynes Convention Center and make deposits to hold at least 8,000 rooms at Boston's five largest hotels. The HAI had already hired an executive director, Alan Fein, who had considerable experience in personnel and financial management. We also hired staff to organize local meetings, keep records, and prepare a newsletter.

We heard that our application to host the 1992 conference had been approved, just before the occurrence of the San Francisco meeting in the summer of 1990, and we then took our entire staff to learn the essentials of what we must do in Boston 2 years later. My counterpart at the University of California at San Francisco (UCSF) Medical School, who was chair of the 1990 conference, was Dr. Paul Volberding, a clinical researcher who had much experience with HIV/AIDS. I knew Paul and felt comfortable asking for his advice. His deputy co-chair was Dr. Robert Wachter, a junior faculty member in the Department of Medicine at UCSF. The San Francisco area had a large population of gay men and a major epidemic of HIV/AIDS that was overwhelming the city in the 1980s.[56] The Bay Area also had a large number of intelligent, well-informed AIDS activists. Only New York had a comparable contingent of gay activists who were aggressively challenging the medical and political establishments with their protests.

Alan, Yamil, and I were pleased to see the apparent success of the San Francisco conference. Although there were many protests outside the hall, they were handled with little or no violence, and the scientific sessions seemed to go on without disruption. That changed, however, on the last day of the meeting when Dr. Louis Sullivan, Bush's secretary of health and human services, spoke about the governmental approach to AIDS at the final plenary session. More than 1,000 protesters were strategically placed at the front of the large conference room. Soon after Dr. Sullivan began speaking, he was barraged with objects thrown at him, heckled, and soon completely drowned out with noise from whistles and horns. No one was seriously injured, but it was clear that the protesters had blocked him from delivering his message.

As our Harvard team discussed these matters with our UCSF friends, it was clear that they expected turmoil and were somewhat relieved that the only major disruption was at the talk of Dr. Sullivan. Drs. Volberding and Wachter impressed upon us the importance of including AIDS activists at all stages of the planning for the upcoming Boston conference. We established a strong relationship with Larry Kessler, the founding director of the AIDS Action Committee (AAC) of Massachusetts. The AAC worked closely with the Fenway Community Health Clinic, which at the time provided clinical care for the largest number of AIDS patients in the Boston area. Larry suggested that we appoint local activists to all the committees we had organized to prepare for the conference. We did, and the community advisors usually provided good advice. But as we soon learned, all the heavyweight AIDS activists for the East Coast were in New York and largely disconnected from their counterparts in Boston.

Bob Wachter, the co-chair of the San Francisco conference, strongly advised us to hire a director for community relations, someone who was trusted by the AIDS activists, so we did. Wachter, who wrote a book about his experience with the activists in San Francisco, specifically suggested Dana Van Gorder, who had served in that role for the San Francisco conference.[146] We hired Dana, initially on a 6-month contract. Dana seemed like a nice fellow, and it was clear that he had many years of experience of community organizing in the San Francisco Bay Area. We'd soon learn that this didn't count for much with the East Coast activists, especially the New Yorkers who were the national leaders.

Dana told us our first priority to work with the AIDS activists should be to meet with Larry Kramer and get his blessing. We followed this advice and took a trip to Manhattan to meet Kramer at his apartment. We introduced ourselves and explained our mission, which was to work with him and the activists to have a productive conference in Boston. Larry made a joke about a foul odor in his apartment. "I just can't get rid of that smell," he said. "It comes from the flat below. Ed Koch [the previous mayor of New York City] lives there." He went on about how he respected me and would help us with the meeting, briefing the AIDS activist leaders in the New York community. He then said, "The first thing you have to do is to get rid of this f--ker," pointing at Dana Van Gorder, who had brought us there. "He is nothing but trouble." We were flabbergasted and embarrassed as we came back to Boston. I never did understand why Kramer was against Van Gorder. I had several phone conversations with Kramer after I got home, including one when he wanted me to join a protest against President Bush in Kennebunkport. I politely declined. Some of my Boston friends who knew Kramer warned me about getting too close to him, that he was "unpredictable and dangerous." But in my talks with Larry, he taught me much about the discrimination and hate that was so often directed at AIDS patients.

Over the winter and spring, we spent a considerable amount of time meeting with the various committees we had set up, meeting with activists, and talking with the folks who had organized the San Francisco conference as well as a few of the Italians who were organizing the Florence conference that would occur in 1991. One of the senior officials organizing the Florence conference was Dr. Gino Chieco-Bianchi, a former dean of medicine at the University of Padua and a dear friend. I first met Gino in 1971, when I was a postdoctoral fellow in Europe, and much later, he spent a sabbatical year in my lab. I knew he'd give me any inside information he had about problems they had in organizing the meeting, like how to get funding from the WHO. So in June 1991, our group departed for Florence, hoping we could learn enough to put on a successful meeting in Boston the following year.

chapter twenty-three

Protests in Italy

We left for Florence, Italy, determined to learn as much as possible about the rapidly changing politics of AIDS. While that wasn't on our radar when we first bid to host the conference 2 years earlier, it now seemed essential to prepare for a peaceful meeting in Boston. Along with Alan Fein, our executive director, and Yamil Kouri, I traveled with Drs. Ric Marlink and Phyllis Kanki, who were former trainees in my lab and close friends. They were now junior faculty members at Harvard. Upon arrival in Florence, Ric, Phyllis, and I met with Christopher Sands to hear the scuttlebutt about activists' plans. Christopher was a gay man, a Harvard grad who was well connected in Los Angeles, and a Hollywood writer and producer for 20th Century Fox, ABC, and NBC. At the time of our visit to Hollywood a few years before, Christopher generously agreed to work the Harvard Club of Los Angeles to help the Harvard AIDS Institute with both fundraising and influence. By the time we got to Florence, Christopher had become a trusted advisor.

The opening ceremony, which was on June 16, 1991, seemed to portend a difficult week, at least for us. The opening session usually features talks by the organizers, the local politicians, the WHO, and a celebrity or two. The celebrity opener turned out to be President Yoweri Museveni of Uganda. This was a mistake. In one sense it seemed logical, as Uganda was one of the first countries in Africa to experience the devastating HIV epidemic that would later wreak major havoc on most of sub-Saharan Africa. But Museveni was also one of the African leaders who blamed the high-risk groups from the north, like gay men, for supposedly bringing the HIV virus to Africa. This was proven to be untrue, as the A and D viruses of Uganda were different from the HIV-1B that caused the epidemic in the United States and Europe. But autocrats often pay little heed to science or logic, and Museveni had a bad record on human rights, especially with the LGBTQ population. He is still in power after about 40 years, and his government has passed legislation that prescribes such penalties as up to 20 years in prison for "promotion of homosexuality" and life imprisonment for "homosexual acts."[147]

By the middle of the week, it was clear that the AIDS activists were riled up. The number of participants in "die-in" type protests, where a protester lies down next to a cut-out gravestone and pretends to be dead, kept increasing. Of equal importance, the activists were condensing and clarifying their message. They were also becoming more aggressive.

On the afternoon of Wednesday, June 19, we held an open meeting where we explained our plans for the 1992 meeting in Boston. Seated on the stage with Yamil and I were about 10 others who would take responsibility for inviting speakers in the different areas of AIDS science, as well as senior representatives from the US CDC, the World Health Organization, and the International AIDS Society. The room we had reserved held only 300 people, but it was full. About 50 were protesters. The purpose of the session was to give an overview of our plans for the Boston meeting, to encourage questions, and to solicit advice from interested parties. It was soon clear that the protesters were dominating the dialogue. For many of us, it was clear that they had their own agenda.

Some of their agenda items were quite logical and not difficult for us to fulfill, like updates on drug trials and how to better exchange information with community organizations. But it was soon apparent that one issue was about something over which we had no control. It was the policy adopted by the Reagan and then the Bush White House, which stated that HIV-positive people who were not US citizens would not be allowed to enter the country to attend the meeting. We made it very clear that we thought that

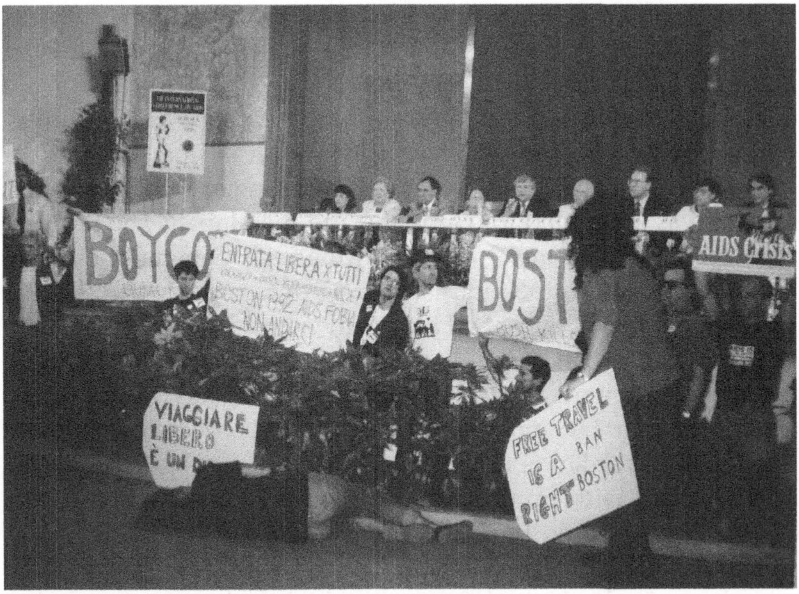

Figure 23.1: Protests against plans for Boston AIDS conference

policy was wrong, and we would do all we could to get our government to change the policy. Several people, both activists and scientists, offered to help us organize letter campaigns and meetings with US Congresspeople. Seated on the stage, just to my left, was Dr. Jonas Salk, who had become famous for making the first polio vaccine. I knew Jonas fairly well, so I asked him if he could help us. He said he probably could, that he knew Bush, but he could only be effective if he did it behind the scenes, away from the public approaches. He said he'd try to get a meeting at the White House and would bring me with him. That didn't happen.

By Thursday, it was clear that we were in a tough spot. On Friday, I would have to give a speech about the upcoming Boston meeting, about how all would be warmly welcomed to our great city. Some important organizations, like the San Francisco AIDS Foundation and the International AIDS Society (IAS), stated that they would not endorse the convening of any international conference on HIV in any country that discriminated against travelers on HIV status. The foundation further stated they would boycott any conferences that took place under such conditions.

The IAS was in fact the major authority under which the international AIDS conferences were held. We, in Boston, weren't the only ones in this plight. After the 1992 meeting in Boston, the conference was scheduled for Germany and then Japan. The meeting held before San Francisco was in Montreal. Canada, Germany, Japan, and many other industrialized democracies had similar restrictions against entry by HIV-positive noncitizens.

Some pragmatists pointed out that a distinction should be made between restrictions for travel to the United States versus immigration. Foreign HIV-positive travelers would be less likely to pose the potential burden of long-term health-care expenses that might be associated with immigration. It was clear that no one in the United States should be afraid of HIV-infected foreigners unless they planned to have sex or share needles with them. In fact, HIV prevalence in the United States was higher than in most other countries, so potential partners from the United States were more likely to infect outsiders than were visitors from other countries to infect Americans.

We had more meetings with activists and IAS officials. We were told that Mother Teresa, who was scheduled to speak just before me in the final session, had to cancel because she couldn't get out of Iraq. The activists made it clear that they would close down a meeting in Boston with violent protests. As the night wore on, I huddled with Ric Marlink, Phyllis Kanki, and Christopher Sands to prepare my speech for the next morning. I knew I had to be clear and frank, but I also had to vent my anger. Christopher used his Hollywood writing skills to sharpen my statements. We called John Shattuck, a vice president at Harvard, to explain the dilemma, that the millions Harvard had already invested would probably be lost. We were lucky to have Shattuck as our point person. He was a legal scholar who would soon go on to become the assistant Secretary of State for Democracy and Human Rights in the Clinton administration.

As the morning began, I steeled myself to rise to the occasion. It turned out to be the most memorable speech of my career. It was evident that the audience in the conference hall was tense. Hundreds of activists were lined up in front, ready to pounce. I had been up all night, but adrenaline and anger kept me alert. So at 11 am, just before the scheduled ending of the Italy conference, I delivered the following speech.

> I have thrown out my original speech. I have stayed up most of the night preparing another. Please listen.
>
> A journalist said to me yesterday that I had made a non-statement regarding whether the Boston conference would take place as scheduled. Let me change that impression.
>
> There will be no conference in Boston next year unless all American travel and immigration restrictions against HIV-infected people are lifted by August 3rd.
>
> As a scientist, I had never expected to be so preoccupied with the issue of national politics. I admit I was naive.
>
> At Wednesday's press conference, my inability to successfully navigate between the activists and the journalists was apparent.
>
> I know in my heart, however, that the world will be ill-served by the loss of international communication. The cooperation that will be blocked if the Bush administration does not change its misguided and discriminatory travel and immigration policies will be a major setback for all of us.
>
> But let me be blunt. Science must be honest and so will I.
>
> There are two issues at play here – restrictions against travel by the HIV-infected and those of immigration. There is a broad range of diverse opinion. The IAS, the WHO, and the National Commission on AIDS state that they would support the Boston conference if travel restrictions alone are lifted. The Gay Men's Health Crisis Center and ACT UP have made clear their threats to disrupt and shut down a conference that takes place if the travel restriction alone are lifted. All of these organizations have their own agendas.
>
> The mutual respect and coordination required between the communities of activists, PWAs [persons with AIDS], and the local

organizing committees are equally critical in the relationship between the scientific organizing committees and the International AIDS Society.

It may also surprise you to learn that the chairs of the 1991, 1992, and 1993 conferences have no representation on the very organization formed to recognize and coordinate these conferences.

I must apologize to many of the international members of the conference for the parochial and domestic focus of my remarks, but please hear me out.

I am not the smooth politician that some would wish me to be. I am grieved that the crass, domestic American political agenda and the ultimatums I have received from activists have conspired in a bizarre alliance to deny the free exchange of information necessary to fight AIDS.

Make no mistake, the Bush administration does not want an AIDS forum, especially not during the election year of 1992. How ironic, to provide the US right-wing bigots with precisely the outcome they desire.

Well over 100,000 deaths in the United States have been documented. In the US, persons with AIDS have a voice but have not been adequately heard. The Third World, however, is experiencing 95% of all new HIV infections. These people will most certainly die with no voice at all.

We must not be so preoccupied by our own domestic policy problems that we close our minds to their pain and suffering.

And let us acknowledge that the US is not alone in its discriminatory policies. Are we confident that a person with HIV can so freely emigrate to those countries designated as our future sites?

I am not hopeful that there will be a Boston conference. As an American and a scientist, I am outraged at the discriminatory US policies. My staff and I will work tirelessly during the next month and a half to bring our government to its senses. I implore each and every one of you to return to your supportive colleagues, families, and friends armed with more of our letters to send to my government.

We must recapture the spirit we all felt at the opening of the San Francisco Conference. Scientists, people with HIV, health-care professionals, and activists communicating effectively with mutual respect in our common battle.

Please participate in the march to the US Consulate here in Florence – let us make our protest loud and clear to my government.

The threat to our international fight against AIDS from intransigence, belligerence, and the denial of human rights may well leave us without the Boston Conference.

But frankly, however, at least I can return to my research lab. (1st slide, please)

This is Magdalena Bankowski from Switzerland, Boris Renjifo from Colombia, Dieudonne Mubikayi from Zaire, Aissatou Gueye from Senegal, Lukumuena Kashala from Zaire, Xiaofang Yu from China, and Woan-Roah Lee from Taiwan.

These people represent the core, the stimulus, and the intellectual strength of my own AIDS research effort. They are my students, my teachers, my friends. They do not represent politics, ignorance, fear, or confrontation. They represent instead our hope for a future without AIDS. They, more than any words I can offer, best symbolize my vision of a World United Against AIDS.

In any event, let us join together in Dakar, Senegal, for the 6th Annual AIDS in Africa meeting in December.

It is not the loss of Boston that matters ultimately. It is the loss of solidarity, the lack of respect for human rights, and the loss of our rights to the free exchange of ideas that pose such a serious catastrophe for a successful effort against this AIDS pandemic.

Thank you.

As I finished, there was thunderous applause, and the audience of 9,000 or so all stood. We then marched to the US Consulate about a mile away. I was in the front row of marchers. There were hundreds of journalists observing it all. The *New York Times, Wall Street Journal, Washington Post, Boston Globe,* and most other major US news outlets ran the story either that night or the next day. Even when we had had major scientific discoveries, I had tried to avoid the limelight. This time it was impossible.

After asking for permission, the *Washington Post* published my speech.[148] Pat Buchanan, a right-wing extremist presidential candidate, the Rush Limbaugh/Tucker Carlson–type personality of the time, wrote a column about me and the need to stamp out "political correctness." The Family Research Council, which has led on issues like opposition to LGBTQ rights and same-sex marriage, eagerly expressed their support for a travel ban against

HIV-infected foreigners. More than 100,000 letters were sent to the Bush White House to urge a change in policy. We used whatever influence Harvard had to get Secretary of Health and Human Services Lewis Sullivan to change the policy. I published a piece in a leading AIDS journal urging that the exclusionary US policy be changed.[149]

In July, we were told there was a 50–50 chance that HIV would be removed from the list of restrictions against travel and immigration. Eventually, the travel ban would be lifted – in 2010, during the Obama administration. I resigned my position as chair of the conference in early August and stated that the meeting was canceled. The Boston Sheraton and other hotels sued Harvard for loss of income. I gave a deposition. Some leading activists testified about their high degree of confidence that there would have been violence at the conference had it occurred. Harvard lost the case.

Some colleagues at Harvard urged that we negotiate with the Netherlands to run the meeting in Amsterdam instead. I said that arrangement would be fine with me, but I would not agree to chair the conference. I was done with AIDS politics. I just wanted to return to my research. Dr. Jonathan Mann, who had recently come to Harvard after resigning as head of the WHO Global Programme on AIDS, agreed to replace me as chair of the meeting. The conference took place in Amsterdam in the summer of 1992 without any notable disturbances.

In May 1992, at about the same time we had been planning for the AIDS conference in Boston, I was invited to receive an honorary doctorate at the University of Maryland. There were three of us there to receive honorary degrees. One was Sister Mary Thomas, who had been president and CEO of the Mercy Medical Center in Baltimore. The second, seated immediately to my left, was Dr. Louis Sullivan, the secretary of health and human services in the George H.W. Bush administration – the very same person who was the face of the discriminatory HIV restrictions and to whom we had directed our pleas for change. The dean, Dr. Errol Reese, called me first. He mentioned the usual accolades about contributing to finding the cause of AIDS and making a blood test. Beyond these things, he went on to say, "Although he is a scientist, Dr. Essex showed the courage to speak out against his government when their policies discriminated against people with HIV/AIDS." Apparently, he didn't realize that my criticisms and protest had been directed at Dr. Sullivan, who was next up to be recognized.

I later learned, however, that Dr. Sullivan wasn't the real villain of the discriminatory policy. It was Richard Thornburgh, Bush's attorney general. Apparently Sullivan had spoken in favor of lifting the travel ban, but Thornburgh was strongly opposed, and Bush went with Thornburgh.

chapter twenty-four

Development and Deeda Blair

All who are involved with financial or administrative matters at Harvard are familiar with the phrase "each tub on its own bottom." What it means is that each of the 12 schools must raise sufficient funds to balance their own budget. The revenue comes principally from four sources: tuition, endowment, targeted research support, and gifts for current use. The targeted research support is primarily grants or contracts from the US government, especially the NIH, but a small fraction is from established foundations such as the American Cancer Society. For the university as a whole, and the Faculty of Arts and Sciences, which includes the undergraduate college, only about 20% of operating costs come from student tuition. This means that many students, especially the undergraduates, are on partial or full financial scholarship. It allows Harvard to accept and enroll exceptionally talented students from anywhere in the world, independently of the applicant's ability to pay.

Harvard University has an endowment in excess of $50 billion, which is the largest among US universities. For the fund to grow in perpetuity at a robust level, it is invested in such a way that the annual "payout" is usually only 3–4%. Though the entire endowment is managed as one total pool of money, it is actually composed of many different funds that are owned by the different faculties or schools and even particular departments within the schools.

For the Harvard T.H. Chan School of Public Health (HSPH), only about 20% of the annual income is from endowment. The majority, about 60%, is from grants and contracts. This includes a proportion of faculty salaries. As a result, most faculty develop the skills of grantsmanship, if only for self-preservation. The same situation applies for faculty at the Medical School, especially the large number of affiliated faculty based at the Harvard hospitals, where the same general rules apply.

New deans are required to seek donations to their schools, especially unrestricted gifts, and especially to increase the endowment, rather than just to raise funds for annual use. Most faculty, on the other hand, prefer that funds be raised for current use and targeted to their research interests and to the support of graduate students. Deans usually employ a large staff of development officers under an assistant dean for development. In Harvard jargon, the term "development" is a euphemism for fundraising.

The primary target for fundraising is usually alumni. Many alumni of Harvard College are financially secure and therefore obvious targets for development. This is also true for graduates of the Business School. But the premise of "each tub on its own bottom," regarding school funding, has usually been understood as restricting faculty and deans to raising funds from their own alumni. This poses challenges for the HSPH. Dean Harvey Fineberg used to say to students at the time of commencement that "you are the only group who will make less money after graduation than you did before you enrolled." This is so because many HSPH students are physicians or other professionals who will become public health officials in government or academia after graduation. So HSPH alumni are not a group that would normally be suitable as large donors. To get around this, magnanimous deans or presidents sometimes allow or even encourage groups such as College or Business School alumni to make donations to the poorest tubs like the School of Education or HSPH.

When potential donors have topics of personal interest, such as cancer, AIDS, or global warming, they may identify specific schools or faculty members as most appropriate for their gifts. Indeed, many "targeted donors" are not Harvard alumni. They just want to support a cause and may feel that scientists doing research at places like Harvard are more likely to be successful. This can create competition among deans, development officers, and faculty members who may already be known to potential donors. One head of development at HSPH, who had just moved into the position, commented to me on how different this was from her former institution, the Perkins School for the Blind in Watertown, Massachusetts. At the Perkins School, she said, "all faculty there are unified around the same cause, to educate the children." She was right. I know the Perkins School well, as my sister, Cynthia Essex, was there for her 50-year career, first as a teacher and later as head of the Lower School. But Harvard is a very different environment, especially at the graduate schools, where faculty may be in stiff competition for resources needed to conduct their research.

Deeda Blair, who was a co-chair of the International Advisory Council for the Harvard AIDS Institute (HAI), was indefatigable at raising funds for our AIDS research and, thankfully, hugely successful. She and her husband Bill were long-standing supporters of liberal causes, having been introduced to the political and social arena by leaders of the Democratic Party. Bill had been an important diplomat in the 1960s. After deciding to investigate African HIVs, we looked for an introduction to government officials in Senegal who might endorse our research. Bill connected us with his law partner, David Morse, who had been director-general of the International Labor Organization and had won the Nobel Peace Prize with that group in 1969. He introduced us to Abdou Diouf, the president of Senegal. Diouf even joined the International Advisory Council of HAI.

Deeda was an early deputy of Mary Lasker, who was probably the single most important lobbyist and fundraiser for medical research in the United States for about three decades. Mary's mobilization of societal and business leaders was probably the pre-eminent reason for a massive expansion of the NIH in the 1960s and 1970s, and for successfully funding the American Cancer Society. Deeda was a major force in her own right, raising money for cancer, neurological diseases, and the NIH. As AIDS became the cause of the 1980s, she became laser-focused on AIDS.

After I shared the Lasker Prize for HIV/AIDS, I was the major beneficiary of her efforts. The prize was shared by Bob Gallo, Luc Montagnier, and myself. She couldn't do much to help Gallo,

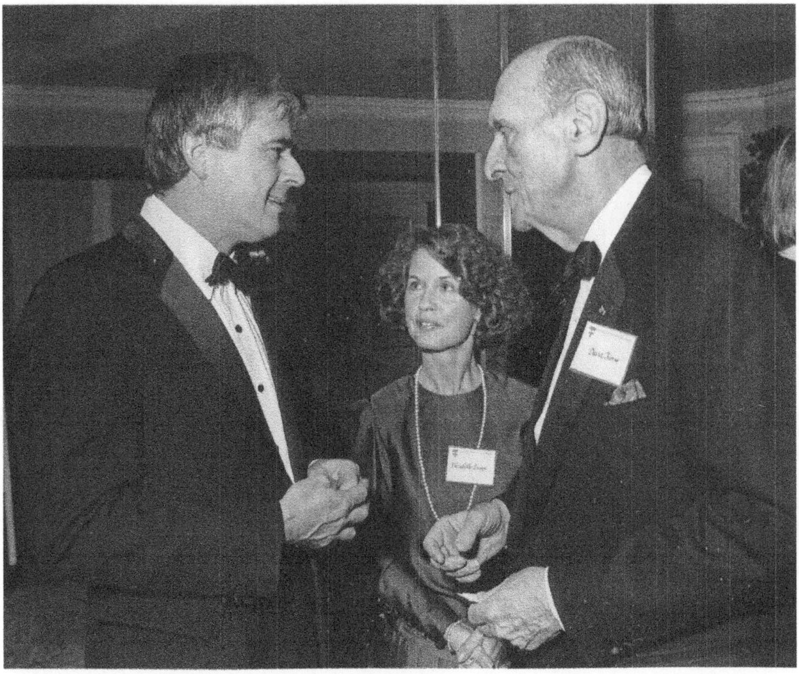

Figure 24.1: Max Essex, Elizabeth Essex, David Morse

because he was at the NIH, or Montagnier, because he was in France. That left me as the most obvious recipient.

Deeda knew I went to the NIH in Bethesda often for committee activities and regularly offered to arrange lunches or dinners at her Washington home with donor prospects or other influential people when I was available. One time, she arranged a dinner for me to meet Ronald Lauder, the son of Estée Lauder of the cosmetics fortune. That morning, she called to say Lauder had to cancel at the last minute. Deeda then said, "Don't worry, come anyway, I'll find someone to join us." When I arrived that evening, Deeda said, "I found someone." It was Katharine Graham, the tycoon publisher of the *Washington Post* and, at the time, one of the most sought-after dinner guests in Washington.

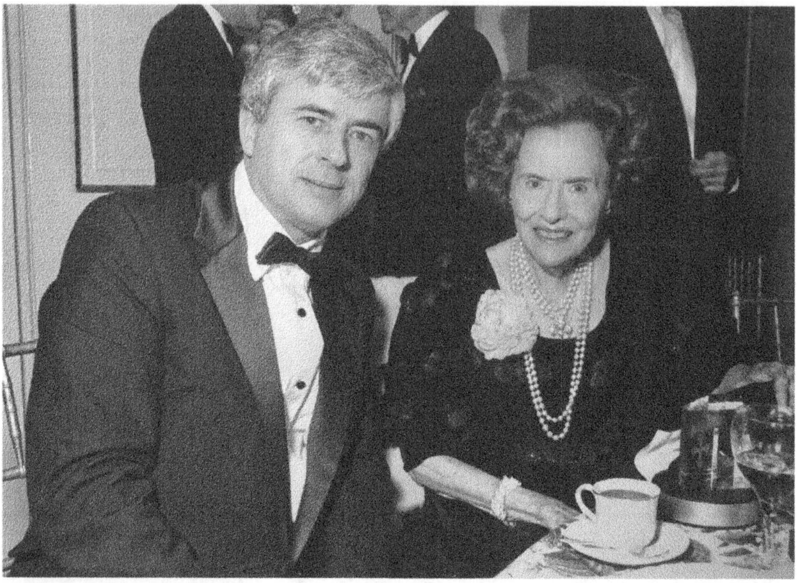

Figure 24.2: Max Essex, Mary Lasker

On another occasion, Deeda asked if I had adequate access to the Massachusetts Congressional delegation. It was during Reagan's second term, when there were stirrings about Congress supporting AIDS research, even if Reagan didn't. "We know Tip O'Neill," she said. "He probably needs advice about AIDS." O'Neill was speaker of the House of Representatives from 1977 to 1987 and from Massachusetts. Again, Deeda said, "Give me some dates when you could meet him." I did. When I arrived about 6 weeks later at her home, O'Neill was there with the entire Congressional delegation from Massachusetts, 10 as I recall. We spent the evening talking about the need for research funding.

Deeda then introduced me to two major foundations at a time when they were just beginning to define their interests. Two members of the newly formed board of the Mathers Foundation, James Handelman and John Young, were friends of hers. The foundation was interested in the use of molecular biology to solve medical problems. We were in a good position to respond. We applied for a grant and were successful. It was followed by several renewals. This support came at a time when the NIH had not yet received adequate resources for the AIDS problem.

The Oak Foundation would become even more important. It was established by Alan Parker, a businessman who was born and raised in Zimbabwe, then called Rhodesia. Joshua Ruch, a co-founder of Rho Capital Partners, introduced Deeda to Alan Parker, and Deeda then introduced me to Alan. Alan was a major partner of Duty-Free, an international chain of shops based at major airports. The Oak Foundation was established when he sold about a billion dollars' worth of shares in the company. Although the major focus of the foundation was the environment, they also had an interest in helping Zimbabwe and in HIV/AIDS.

At this time, the early 1990s, Zimbabwe was a mess. The president, Robert Mugabe, had been a leader of the revolution that established the country, but he was eventually ousted as a corrupt dictator who destroyed the national economy. In Zimbabwe and most of southern Africa, HIV was spreading very rapidly. During the 1970s and 1980s, the country had one of the best records for higher education in Africa, especially in medicine. Quite a few Zimbabweans even found their way to Harvard.

We organized a proposal to the Oak Foundation that would support some of our research on AIDS in Africa, while also training AIDS experts from Zimbabwe. The training would be done both in Boston and at our research facility in Botswana. This also served multiple needs. Many young Zimbabweans had migrated to Botswana looking for work, and Botswana desperately needed medical staff to respond to the AIDS epidemic.

We soon filed an application with Oak and received substantial funding. In the early days, the foundation board was composed primarily of members of the Parker family, especially the three children of Alan and Jette. I was often invited to make a presentation, and this was usually followed by a dinner with the family, where even the grandchildren were present. It was a delightful experience. One of the only early members of the Oak board who was not from the family was Bill Cotter, a Harvard Law School graduate who was then president of Colby College. Bill was also a friend of Derek Bok, who was president of Harvard but had previously been dean of the Law School, where he had known Cotter. Derek put in a good word for me. The Oak funding would become instrumental for establishing the Botswana Harvard Partnership.

In the mid- to late 1980s, our research began to generate considerable attention in the press. My natural reaction was to avoid publicity, as it seemed to elicit jealousy among some of my peers and risk misrepresentation or overinterpretation of some of our research findings. But I also recognized the need to disseminate new knowledge about important clinical developments to people who desperately needed help with the AIDS problem. The attention sometimes also led to immediate donations. Soon after getting the Lasker Award, I received a donation of $25,000 in the mail from Joseph Brooks, a person I had never heard of. In an accompanying note, Brooks mentioned that he had multiple friends and employees with AIDS and just wanted to support research on the topic. Eventually, I got to know Joe and his family. He was chair and CEO of the Lord and Taylor and Ann Taylor clothing chains.

Howard Hiatt, my former dean, also introduced me to Irene Diamond, who had recently set up the Aaron Diamond Foundation in memory of her husband. She invited me to submit an application and then provided research support to our lab for several years. Subsequently, the foundation established the Aaron Diamond AIDS Research Center in New York City and recruited Dr. David Ho as director. Ho became a popular figure in 1996 when he was designated *Time*'s "Person of the Year." We knew David well. He trained at Harvard, primarily with my friend Marty Hirsch, but he had also spent a brief period in my lab learning some techniques.

As a style icon herself, Deeda Blair had many friends in the fashion industry. Among others, she introduced us to Ralph Lauren, Hubert de Givenchy, Princess Ala von Auersperg, Mary McFadden, Gloria Vanderbilt, and Bill Blass. I once attended a small black-tie dinner for Bill Blass in New York, then stuffed my tux into a FedEx box to send home and flew overnight to Japan for a small meeting sponsored by Princess Takamatsu the next day. I began to feel like a real jet-setter.

Deeda also introduced me to Mouna Ayoub, who would later come to the attention of the *New York Times* because of her collection of haute couture.[150] Of Lebanese origin, she married, then divorced, a Saudi prince and moved to Paris. Deeda brought her to visit our lab at Harvard in 1998. While they toured the lab, Mary Fran McLane, our lab manager, explained that we needed a DNA sequencing machine to examine large numbers of HIVs from AIDS patients. "We could do much more if we had one of the new machines," explained Mary Fran. Mouna asked how much the instrument would cost. "About $125,000," said Mary Fran. The next day Mouna gave us a check for the full amount. A month or two later, we got another check from Nasser Al-Rashid, her ex-husband in Saudi Arabia.

Deeda also introduced us to the Prince of Wales Foundation and to quite a few major donors – such as Serge Varsano in Paris, Pierre Durand, Khalil Rizk, Cathy Graham, Elaine Weiler, Howard Slatkin, Arthur Loeb, Dwayne Andreas, John McFadden, Waring Hopkins, Judy Peabody, and Barry Diller – and to Kate and Tod Sedgwick, who became friends of Elizabeth and myself. We were similarly introduced to Richard Smith, the editor-in-chief of *Newsweek*, and his wife, Dr. Soon-Young Yoon, a Harvard-trained anthropologist. Both Ric and Soon-Young have generously helped me and others at HAI with our writing.

Our local group of Harvard-based alumni and friends was also instrumental in the development of HAI. They included Bruce Beal, Esmond Harmsworth, Susan Curren, Jim and Joanne Moore, B Wu and Eric Larson, Dorothy Ganick, Ardie Rodale, Alan Aisenberg, and Julie and Bayard Henry.

In 1999, we had a large benefit dinner at the Plaza Hotel in New York to celebrate the tenth anniversary of HAI. Kofi Annan, the secretary-general of the United Nations, was the featured speaker. Of particular importance, we gave awards to Deeda Blair, Marguerite Littman, and Judy Peabody for all they had done to help us and to alleviate suffering from the AIDS epidemic.

Deeda also introduced me to Maurice Tempelsman, who would have a profound impact on our ability to do AIDS research in Africa. Maurice was born in Belgium and came to the United States as a child. He was a longtime companion of Jacqueline Kennedy Onassis and chair of Lazar Kaplan, the largest diamond company in the United States. He has a long-standing interest in Africa and much experience in diplomacy with African leaders. In the mid-1980s, when our HIV research led us to explore the African epidemic, I explained our needs to Deeda. Our needs included some funding, because at the time, the NIH had only meager funding for AIDS and nothing for Africa. Deeda introduced me to Maurice in the mid-1980s, asking if he knew of any foundations or people who might support our exploratory research in Senegal. Maurice said, "Oh, Deeda, I'll do it." It was our first substantial donation for the research. Maurice also became a valued personal friend who would become instrumental in our research in Africa for the next 35 years.

chapter twenty-five

On to Botswana

By the mid-1990s, it was apparent that a new and more aggressive epidemic of HIV/AIDS was taking place in southern Africa, particularly the region south of Congo and Kenya. Countries like Zambia, Zimbabwe, Botswana, Namibia, and Swaziland (now called Eswatini) were experiencing very high rates of new infections. It was similar for the eastern regions of the Republic of South Africa. The epidemic was clearly due to heterosexual transmission. At least as many women were infected as men. The impact of homosexual transmission seemed to be negligible. Blood transmission by transfusions or dirty needles also seemed to be minimal. Blood screening tests were available. They worked fine, and they were usually used.

The new epidemic seemed similar to the epidemic in Thailand, but much larger. It was even more ominous than the earlier epidemics in Uganda and Central Africa. In most countries of southern Africa, 20% or more of adults were infected. I decided that our research group should get involved to try to understand what was going on. Was it a new and different HIV?

At the time, our research group had extensive interactions in Asia and other parts of Africa but none in southern Africa in the most affected countries. My analysis of the situation suggested that we should consider several issues before deciding on a specific site for collaboration. The most obvious was to select a country with one of the highest rates of infection. For intervention trials, the results come in more quickly if large numbers of people can be rapidly enrolled. Another consideration would be to choose

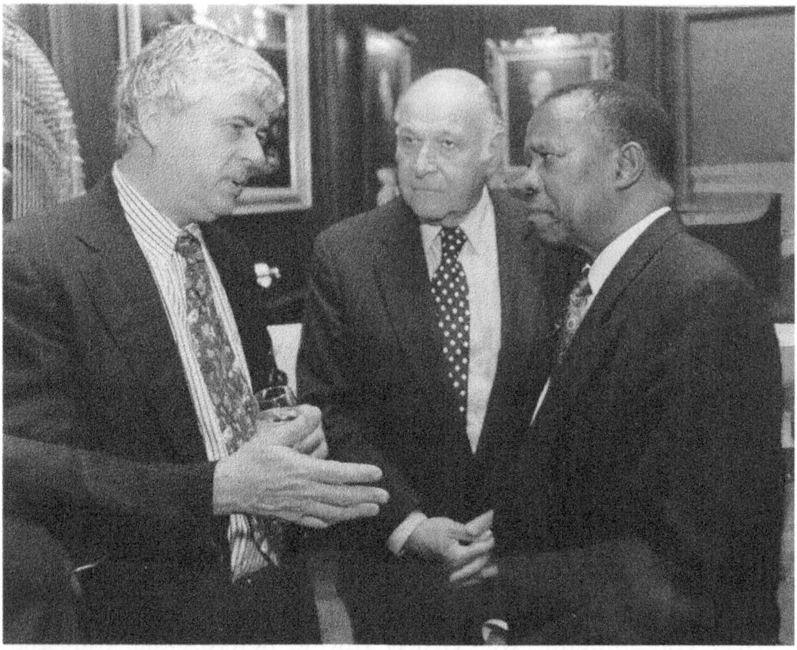

Figure 25.1: Max Essex, Maurice Tempelsman, President Quett Masire

a country where the government was stable and likely to be so for the next 10–20 years. If we made a major investment in people and resources, we'd need confidence that the same leaders would still be in positions of influence in the long-term future. A third consideration would be that the government and the health-care sector of the country would be welcoming of outside advice and collaboration. We knew that major prevention or treatment trials could take many years, and we'd have to learn more about the virus and the local epidemic before we could even begin.

I went to see my friend Maurice Tempelsman, whose advice would be invaluable, in June of 1996. As frequently happened when I went to New York, we shared a long and delicious lunch in his dining room. He suggested Botswana or Namibia. He said both were well governed, and the economic situation was good in both countries. I then selected Botswana. According to UNAIDS numbers, HIV rates were a bit higher there, in fact the highest for any country in the world. Maurice said he was co-hosting a dinner in Washington for Quett Masire, the president of Botswana, in a

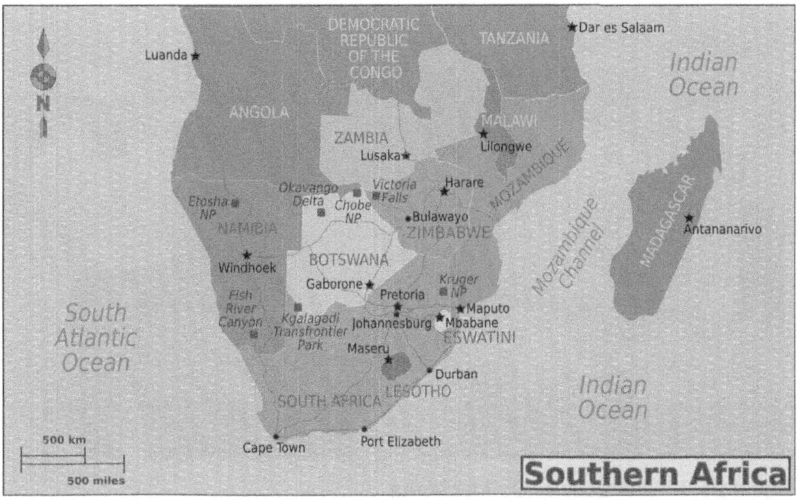

Figure 25.2: Map of Southern Africa
Map by Burmesedays, minor amendments by Joelf – Own work based on the earlier map by Shaund and Nick Roux, CC BY-SA 3.0, https://commons.wikimedia.org/w/index.php?curid=22747926.

few weeks, and he would see that I received an invitation. I got the invitation and attended the dinner.

President Masire was minister of finance for the country soon after it was founded in 1966 and their longest-serving president, in office from 1980 to 1998. He has been described as one of the best postcolonial African leaders for his economic management and his policies on investment in education and health.[151] Soon after the country became independent of Britain in 1966, diamonds would be discovered. As a result, Botswana would go from being one of the poorest countries in Africa to become a middle-income country within two to three decades. Botswana is landlocked, surrounded by Namibia to the west, Zimbabwe to the east, and the Republic of South Africa to the south. Most of Botswana is the Kalahari Desert, with villages and small cities concentrated along the eastern side. The country soon became a destination for high-end safari tourism, having large populations of elephants and other popular wildlife species.

As I arrived at the dinner in Washington, I was introduced to President Masire and Lady Masire in the reception line, but there were many people at the dinner so we didn't have much time to

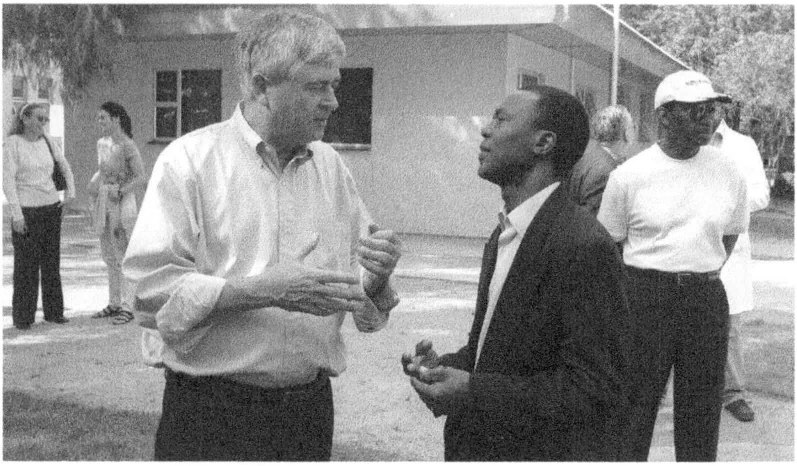

Figure 25.3: Max Essex, Joe Makhema
Photo by Richard Feldman.

talk. I found my seat, which was at one of the last tables in a corner. About halfway through the dinner, I felt a tap on my shoulder. I stood up, turned around, and was surprised to find that it was President Masire. He said, "We need to talk, can we meet for breakfast?" I said, "I really want to talk but I'm scheduled to teach tomorrow morning, in Boston, and am booked on a 6 am flight." He said, "How about tonight right after the dinner? You can ride with me back to my hotel." I said, "Great, I'll meet you right after the dinner." After we arrived at his hotel, he released others in his entourage and asked that I accompany him to meet Dr. Joe Makhema. I learned that Makhema was his physician and major consultant on medical matters. He had not been at the dinner. It was then about 11:30 pm.

President Masire knocked on Makhema's door, obviously waking him up. Dr. Makhema greeted us in his pajamas. President Masire introduced us and stated that he was inviting me to come to Botswana as soon as possible to consult about HIV/AIDS.

President Masire and I soon became friends. I visited with him on most of the trips I made to Botswana during the early years.

My wife and I also got to know his wife Gladys and some of his children, meeting them either at his home or at a local restaurant. On one of their trips to the United States, President Masire and his wife came for a visit at our home outside Boston. We were not accustomed to hosting such high-profile visitors, but his security officers seemed content to leave him alone while they watched television in another room. After Masire left office in 1998, he became a diplomat for various UN peace missions. On one occasion, I met him by chance at a dinner in Abuja, Nigeria, that Dr. Phyllis Kanki of our group had organized with the Nigerian president, Olusegun Obasanjo. On another occasion, I met Masire, again by chance, at a small, isolated inn where he was working on a peace agreement between the leaders of Congo and Angola. He said he needed a break from the tense negotiations so could we just talk and laugh for a while? I loved his warmth and good humor. The last time I saw President Masire was at a celebration of his 90th birthday in 2016. He died a year later and was buried at his home village of Kanye, where he had begun as a farmer.[151]

My first trip to Botswana was about a month after I met President Masire and Dr. Makhema, in August of 1996. I asked Dr. Ric Marlink, the most senior clinical expert in our group, to join me. We took the 17-hour flight from New York to Johannesburg, South Africa, and then a short flight to Gaborone, the capital and the largest city in Botswana. I'd eventually get used to these flights, doing about 100 more over the next 25 years. We were met at the airport by Ria Madison. Ria worked for a Tempelsman diamond processing facility in Molepolole, a town about an hour away from Gaborone. We were then introduced to Jim Barnes, Ria's boss. Barnes worked for Maurice in Botswana and in several other African countries as well. He was a large, gruff man who became much more friendly as you got to know him. He said that Ria was available to help us get around during the time we were there. Maurice then told me that he could make her available a day or two a week to organize things for us after we left.

We met with several other people in Gaborone. In addition to President Masire and Dr. Makhema, they included Joy Phumaphi, the minister of health, John Mulwa, the permanent secretary for health, and Dr. Howard Moffat, who was head of Princess Marina Hospital, the largest hospital in the country. We also met with Sarah Gaolekwe, who was head of the blood bank at the hospital. Dr. Joe Makhema, the president's physician, was also chief of medicine at the hospital, and we would see him in that capacity soon.

Our goal for the first visit was to get a better understanding of the epidemic, to build long-term relationships with local leaders, and to get 15–20 blood samples from infected people to analyze. We succeeded. Our first stop was the Princess Marina Hospital. Joe Makhema took us to a large ward that had eight late-stage AIDS patients in beds and another six on the floor. It was sobering. Joe and Ric took blood samples from the patients and handed them to me to prepare for transport back to Boston. We then went to see a group of patients with sexually transmitted diseases. They, too, were HIV infected, but not yet at a terminal stage of the disease. Our next stop was the blood bank. Sarah Gaolekwe showed us her recent results for the HIV testing of donated blood. From a batch of about 30 samples tested earlier in the week, almost half were positive. It was shocking. Before leaving, we signed an agreement between the government of Botswana and the Harvard AIDS Institute to develop a collaborative research program on HIV/AIDS. We promised to return as soon as we had analyzed virus from the blood samples we obtained.

We brought back samples from 18 patients. Dr. Makhema and his colleagues in Gaborone, Molepolole, and Mochudi would soon collect samples from about 35 additional patients and send them to us in Boston. Soon we had grown viruses in culture from many patients. More than 50 of the viruses were completely sequenced or decoded to reveal every one of the 10,000 letters of their genome. With this information, we learned that the virus causing the epidemic was HIV-1 subtype C, which was quite different from the virus that caused the earlier epidemics in Africa and different from the virus causing the epidemics in the United States, Thailand, and Europe.

It was soon apparent that HIV-1C was spreading so fast that it now caused more than half of the world's infections. From work done in my lab by Drs. Monty Montano and Vlad Novitsky, two postdoctoral fellows, we also learned that HIV-1C seemed to undergo a higher rate of mutation, or genomic variation, than other HIVs.[152] We also found that the Botswana HIV-1C was hypersensitive to substances released by inflammation. And unlike other HIVs, it appeared that the C virus always entered human cells by a particular co-receptor called CCR5. Virtually all sexual infections with HIV are dependent on this route of entry, whereas blood infections are not. We used this information to evaluate the efficiency of drug treatment, to begin designing experimental vaccines, and to design trials to see if we could reduce mother-to-infant transmissions. The need for the latter seemed acute, as prevalence data indicated that more than a third of the pregnant women in the country were already infected.

At the time we were beginning the studies in Botswana, we had already been doing some research in Tanzania, based in Dar es Salaam, with Drs. Wafaie Fawzi and David Hunter, Harvard epidemiologists who were doing studies there. Tanzania is in East Africa but also at the top of southern Africa. It appeared that the earlier epidemic of HIV-1A and D that had moved down from Uganda and Kenya was beginning to fuse with a newer epidemic of HIV-1C from the south.[119] We found some women who had apparently been infected with two different HIVs, such as A and C. The infants born to these mothers were often infected with a new hybrid virus that was a recombinant, having pieces of genes from both parental viruses.

By the late 1990s, the research done by our group and others showed that several different epidemics were going on in Africa.[153,154] Uganda, perhaps the country most severely hit in East Africa, had peaked at about 12–15% in the early 1990s. By the late 1990s, that epidemic caused by HIV-1A and D had plateaued and gone down in prevalence. The Democratic Republic of Congo, representative of Central Africa, had an epidemic that reached 5 or 6% when it plateaued, even though it was apparently caused by the same viruses as the East Africa epidemic. Senegal and most of West Africa had an epidemic of both HIV-2 and HIV-1A/G, a recombinant, but that epidemic usually didn't infect more than 1–3% of adults. North African countries like Morocco or Egypt never did

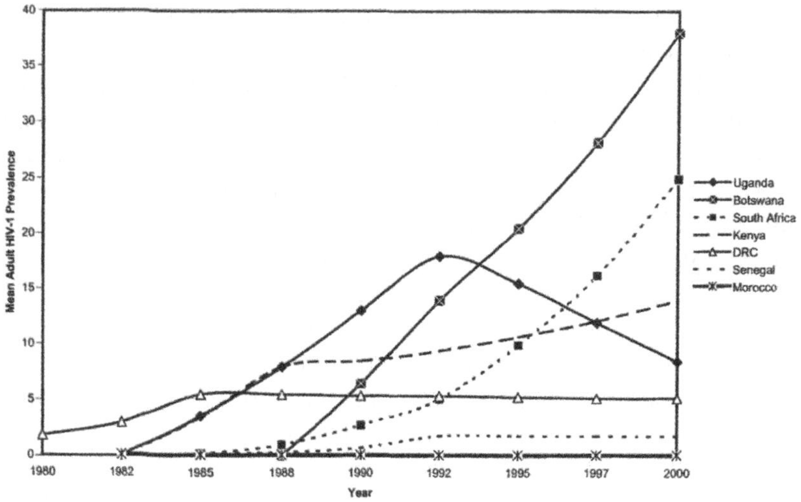

Figure 25.4: Mean adult prevalence rates of HIV for various countries in Africa

Reprinted from Essex M, Mboup S. Regional variations in the epidemic. In: Essex M, Mboup S, Kanki PJ, Marlink RG, Tlou SD, editors. AIDS in Africa. *2nd ed. New York: Kluwer Academic Plenum Publishers; 2002.*

have a serious HIV epidemic. The few cases there appeared to be a spillover from Europe. The more aggressive viruses to the south never seemed to cross the Sahara Desert. So the most transmissible virus was clearly the C of Botswana and the rest of southern Africa. Most of the countries of this region had prevalence rates that were higher than the rates seen anywhere else in the world.

Ric Marlink and I returned to Botswana 3 months after our first visit. We met with several government officials and Drs. Moffat and Makhema to discuss our results. Jim Barnes and Ria Madison took us around town for various meetings and to collect more samples. We consulted with officials from the Ministry of Health to organize a national conference on HIV/AIDS. Many more such meetings and conferences would follow. We talked with Health Minister Phumaphi about increasing our activities in Gaborone and about building a small staff to help with on-site organization. Dr. Moffat at the Princess Marina Hospital said we could use a small storage garage on the hospital grounds. It would be big enough for two or three people with desks and a filing cabinet.

By this time, Ria was spending 2–3 days a week working on our activities. I kept in close touch with Maurice Tempelsman and expressed our gratitude for all he had done through Jim Barnes and Ria, as well as the original help with President Masire. I told Maurice that we hoped to expand rapidly in Botswana, needing two or three full-time people very soon. I said I felt guilty about taking more of Ria's time, as she was trying to juggle our needs with her regular job as personnel manager at the diamond processing plant. Ria mentioned that she'd like to work full time for us but didn't want to put Mr. Tempelsman and Barnes in an awkward position. After more negotiations, Ria became our first employee for the Botswana Harvard Partnership (BHP). She had contacts everywhere in the country and was invaluable to the project. Within 6–8 years, we'd have a staff of more than 300 in the research team on site in Botswana. After 25 years, Ria would still be at BHP.

Our next position would be for someone who was knowledgeable about HIV/AIDS and sensitive enough to represent us with the government and local community leaders. It turned out to be Ibou Thior, a physician from Senegal who was just finishing a graduate degree in epidemiology at Harvard. Ibou was an affable guy who had previously been with us as the head physician for a large cohort of female sex workers exposed to HIV-1 and HIV-2 in Dakar. Ibou's background and qualifications seemed ideal. The Botswana government also helped immensely, providing us with several vehicles and houses for senior staff like Ibou, who were coming from outside the country. To celebrate our progress, Jim Barnes took us for a game drive around Mokolodi, a local reserve that was only about a half-hour from Gaborone. We saw giraffes, kudu, impala, warthogs, wildebeest, a rhinoceros, and many exotic birds. On the way back, we saw a group of baboons around some trash cans at the edge of the city. We were told that leopards sometimes come down from the local hills to catch the baboons.

During the next couple of years, I went back to Botswana often, usually every 2–3 months. Soon it was clear that we needed a

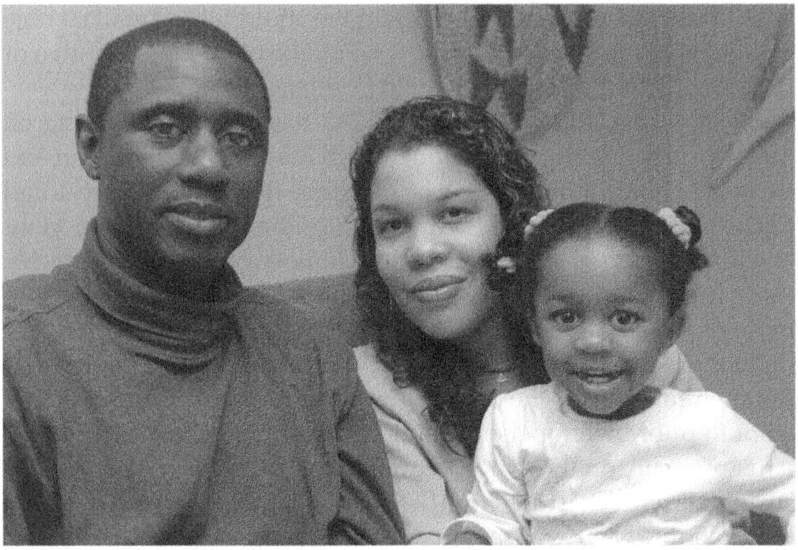

Figure 25.5: Ibou Thior, Tonya Villafana, Aida Thior

research lab at the site. It was inefficient to send samples to Boston for most lab tests, and we had rapidly increasing needs to test new populations. We met with leaders for the national police force, the military, and Debswana, the Botswana national diamond mining company. Norman Moleboge, the head of the police, was welcoming and cooperative. We negotiated an arrangement where we could determine infection rates among police in return for some of our staff providing educational talks about HIV/AIDS at the police academy. We also initiated studies with Debswana, the national diamond company that was formed between De Beers in South Africa and the government of Botswana. Tsetsele Fantan, a senior manager at the company, took us from Gaborone to Jwaneng, the site of the largest diamond mine in the world. I wondered if it might be my last trip as we drove along narrow roads in the Kalahari at speeds well over 100 mph in her Mercedes. The mine was impressive, with the most gigantic trucks I had ever seen moving the alluvia and an exit screening that made the airport TSA checking system look rudimentary. The analysis of blood samples from workers in different job categories showed the lowest rate of HIV infection that we found in Botswana. This might have been because Jwaneng is quite isolated and because the workers, who were considered very valuable, got extensive education on prevention of HIV infection.

Over the next year or two, we continued to expand our activities with the Botswana Harvard Partnership (BHP). Dr. Moffat, the head of Princess Marina Hospital, found a small facility on the hospital campus where we could house four or five lab workers. We hired four local technicians to conduct diagnostic and research tests, and purchased enough equipment so they could function. Dr. Monty Montano, a postdoctoral fellow in our Boston lab, agreed to move to Botswana for 6 months to help get a lab established. When Monty came back, Dr. Sui-yuan Chang, a young Taiwanese woman in our group who had just finished her PhD, offered to go to Gaborone to replace Monty. Both were popular with the Batswana, representing us extremely well. Monty is now a professor at Harvard and Sui-yuan a professor at National Taiwan University. Of the four Batswana technicians we initially hired, two would soon go on to get PhDs themselves. One, Simani Gaseitsiwe, got his PhD from the Karolinska Institute in Stockholm in the same department where I had done postdoctoral training. A third would soon die from AIDS. Hers was the first of the AIDS funerals I attended in Botswana.

As we began to do research with human samples in Botswana, we consulted with the Human Subjects Committee at Harvard to get assurance that our research plans were ethical and beneficial to Botswana. As our research was based at Princess Marina Hospital, a government institution, we also got approval from the Botswana Ministry of Health to do the studies. As the research expanded in Botswana, with plans to include human trials, we worked with Botswana to train health officials on the ethical standards for conducting trials. This included trips to Botswana by the leaders of the Harvard Ethics Committee and extended training in Boston for Botswana health officials to build capacity on research ethics within the country.

In 1998, President Masire would end his term and retire. We would miss Masire's help, but Maurice Tempelsman had already introduced me to Festus Gontebanye Mogae, who was elected to succeed Masire as president, when Mogae was the vice president under Masire. Mogae was trained in economics in the United Kingdom and, several years earlier, had been the minister of finance.

At least once per year, Elizabeth would join me on an African trip so we could take a brief holiday. We'd usually go to a game park in northern Botswana or to a bordering country like Namibia or Zimbabwe. One time, we went to the Chobe Game Lodge, a sumptuous resort near the Zambezi River where Elizabeth Taylor had gone on two of her honeymoons. We saw herds of 30 or more elephants, numerous antelope, hippos, lions, and Cape buffalo. Monkeys ran in the room to steal packets of coffee creamer and sugar if we neglected to latch the door.

By the turn of the century, the Botswana population was understandably pessimistic about their future. The funeral industry was the most rapidly expanding segment of the economy. Stanecki and Walker at UNAIDS published a paper entitled "Current Estimates and Projections for the Epidemic,"[155] where they projected that average life expectancy at birth would drop from 72 to 29 years in a decade in Botswana unless something was done to change the death curves. Fortunately, something was done.

Unity Dow, a justice on the Supreme Court of Botswana, and I wrote a book on the human cost of the epidemic in Botswana.[102] She described the personal anguish and devastation of friends, family, and acquaintances caused by the epidemic, while I provided a medical explanation for each dire outcome. The title *Saturday Is for Funerals* came from the recognition that Saturdays were no longer available for weddings and other celebrations because they were completely consumed by funerals. The book includes chapters on a range of topics from sexual transmission to disease treatment, as experienced by the people of Botswana. The British author Alexander McCall Smith wrote a popular series about Botswana called *The No. 1 Ladies' Detective Agency* featuring a Motswana detective, Mma Precious Ramotswe. One book he wrote later in the series was called *The Saturday Big Tent Wedding Party.*[156] I was honored by the gesture when he dedicated the book to me for the role our group played in contributing to the country's recovery, and Saturdays could return to celebrations.

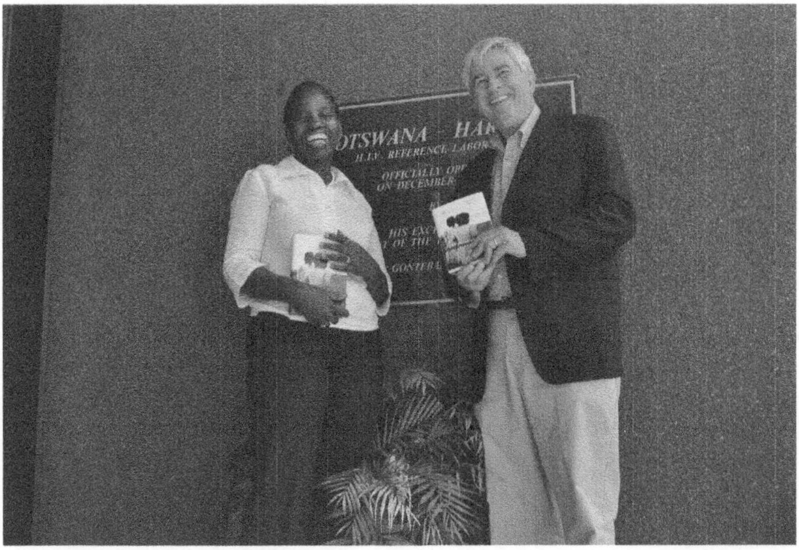

Figure 25.6: Unity Dow, Max Essex

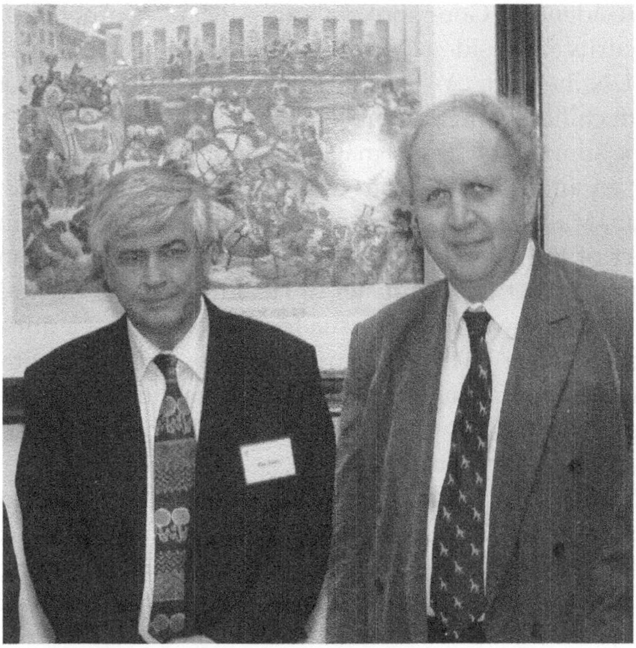

Figure 25.7: Max Essex, Alexander McCall Smith

chapter twenty-six

Saving Children

As the new century began, it was clear that something needed to be done, and fast, to thwart the devastation of HIV/AIDS in southern Africa. Nine countries that collectively had less than 2% of the world's population had the majority of the world's HIV cases. Botswana was at the top of the list. The government, the medical establishment, community leaders, and our Harvard team would all need to do more. In a speech to the UN Security Council, US Vice President Al Gore spoke about AIDS as a problem for war and security.[157] President Mogae certainly did his part. In a speech to the UN, he said, "We are threatened by extinction. People are dying in chillingly high numbers."

In the summer of 2000, I made my first trip to Namibia, following up on an invitation from the country's Prime Minister Hage Geingob. Maurice Tempelsman had introduced me to Geingob at a dinner of the Corporate Council on Africa. The prime minister asked that I meet with Minister of Health Libertina Amathila. My daughter Carrie was in Botswana for the summer as a nurse practitioner volunteer in the pediatric wards, so she went with me to Windhoek. Amathila and the other government officials were welcoming and cooperative. We invited them to visit our program in Botswana, and they did.

By 2000, our research budget was also expanding, allowing us to do more in Africa. Elizabeth also encouraged me to take a sabbatical, so we made plans to move to Botswana. Before going, however, I wanted to set the schedule to complete the second edition of our book *AIDS in Africa*.[79] So with my co-editor Dr. Souleymane Mboup from Senegal and his wife Marie, Elizabeth and I spent the month of October 2000 at the Rockefeller Villa Study Center in Bellagio, on Lake Como in Italy. It is a special place. It brings together scholars from all over the world in a beautiful and luxurious setting. At about the same time we were finalizing the *AIDS in Africa* book, Drs. Vince De Vita, Tony Fauci, myself, and others had just published the fourth edition of *AIDS*, a standard reference book used in the developed world.[142] It was sobering to compare the central questions on treatment for the two reference books. For the AIDS book, written for the United States and other developed countries, there was much recent detail on the use of antiretroviral drugs for the treatment of AIDS patients. The lives of most patients could be saved by using the new drug regimens called HAART for "highly active antiretroviral treatment," which cost $10,000 or more per year. This course of treatment simply wasn't available for most patients in Africa, and most of the patients were in Africa. Many physicians and scientists recognized the gravity of the disparity, and we lobbied all government and pharmaceutical company officials who would listen.

In June 2001, Elizabeth and I left for Botswana. Jim Barnes had recently left the country, and we moved into his former house in Gaborone, which was now available. It was a short walk to our research buildings on the Princess Marina Hospital campus. The chairmanship of our Harvard department would now be assumed by Dr. Tun-Hou Lee during my sabbatical. I'd still come back to Boston for a week or two every 2–3 months, reversing the travel pattern I had previously followed.

For my first trip back to Boston, I left Gaborone in the afternoon of September 10, 2001, connecting in Johannesburg to arrive in New York on the morning of September 11. My flight on South African Airways was one of the last to land before terrorists hit the twin towers of the World Trade Center on their suicide mission. After I arrived, I walked to the next terminal for my brief flight to Boston. As I sat down looking at the large window of the waiting room toward Manhattan, I saw a massive cloud of smoke. Soon after, I saw another. An announcement came over the loudspeaker saying that all flights were canceled, that the airport would close immediately, and that everyone must leave. The airline and concession employees were panicked, running toward the exits, many sobbing. Clearly, they knew more than the passengers like me. I exited the building, deciding I would board the first available ride, which was a shuttle bus for a car rental company. Upon arrival at the car rental headquarters, I was told that no cars were available without reservations. I told the car rental agent the airport was closed, so they could release some cars. They, too, then received an announcement to close but agreed to give me a car just before they did. I drove out of the airport toward the bridges to Connecticut and soon learned from the car radio that all the bridges were closed and more bombings were expected. I then headed east to the end of Long Island. My goal was to get to Orient Point, where a ferry left every hour or so for New London, Connecticut. As I approached the ferry office, I realized that many others had had the same idea. The line of cars waiting to get on was a mile and a half long. I parked, walked to the ferry house, and was told I could get on 30 hours later. I accepted this, booked the reservation, and drove 10 miles back to find a room for the night. I then watched the views of horror as presented by CNN. My daughter Carrie had managed to reach me by cell phone as I left the airport and transmitted the information that I was OK to Elizabeth, who was watching the same events on CNN in Botswana. I got the ferry the next day and drove to Boston, trying to fathom what was going on. After a week, the planes were flying again, and I managed to get back to Botswana. Carrie had a serious boyfriend, Chris, whom I met, and both of them flew back to Botswana with me.

Before I moved to Botswana, I told Minister of Health Joy Phumaphi that our small lab in Gaborone had rapidly become inadequate for all we planned to do. We hoped to start early vaccine trials, adult treatment trials, and large trials to prevent mother-to-child transmission of the virus. Our current space on the Princess Marina Hospital campus was limited to 2,000 square feet between the small lab and two "portacamps" – basic mobile trailers with rooms for office space. Minister Phumaphi assigned one of her deputies, Leonard Manthe, to work with me to develop plans for a new lab building. I told Leonard that we'd need at least 5,000 square feet to allow for imminent expansion. The agreement was that the Botswana government would pay for the building and the Harvard AIDS Institute would provide the staff. Equipping the new lab was also to be a major expense, but we were all greatly relieved to find that the Bill and Melinda Gates Foundation and the Merck Foundation agreed to cover those expenses.

To my great delight, I soon found that both Leonard and Joy Phumaphi were very strong advocates for our building. They said we should go for a much larger facility, perhaps 25,000 square feet. They also said that we should work together to pull out all the stops and have the building done within 6 months. I couldn't believe that was possible but vowed to do all I could to move things along.

Mary Fran McLane, my lab manager in Boston, flew to Botswana with a set of architects' plans that had been used for our lab in Boston. The plans included some rooms that would be classified as biohazard level 3. This is the standard that the US National Institutes of Health (NIH) requires for research done with concentrated samples of dangerous viruses to prevent lab workers from getting infected from the aerosols generated by ultracentrifugation. The Botswana government sought bids from contractors and selected Italaswana, a well-known Italian construction company working in Botswana. They broke ground in July 2001. A schedule was established whereby both Leonard and I would review programs with Italaswana management at least once per month. If the contractor fell more than a month behind, we'd call for a meeting with Minister Phumaphi. If they got even farther behind, she'd call for a meeting with President Mogae. When we threatened the contractor with this, they would greatly expand the crew to speed up, fearful that the government would avoid Italaswana for future projects.

The building was made of brick, and it seemed that most of the heavy work was done by strong women pushing wheelbarrows laden with bricks. Remarkably, the building would be fully erected within 5 months. A celebration was planned for an opening on World AIDS Day, December 1, in 2001. Only one of the three floors was finished, but that was rapidly filled with equipment so tours could be given to show how the lab would function. At 5 am

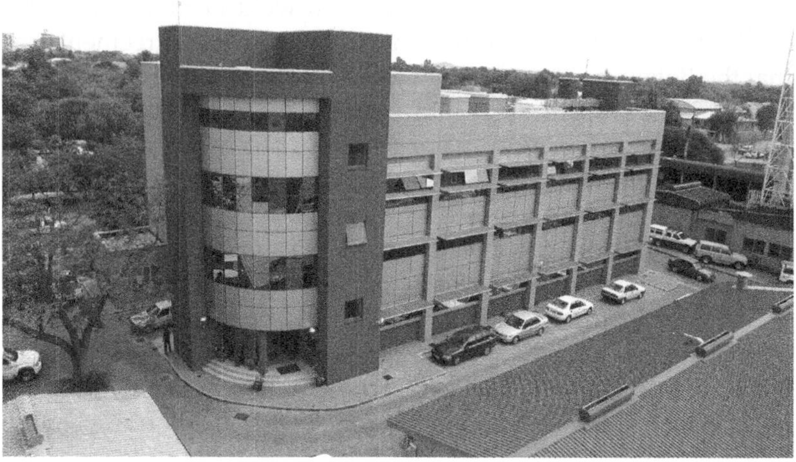

Figure 26.1: Botswana Harvard Partnership Research Laboratory
Photo by Richard Feldman.

on December 1, a huge crew was vigorously working to put in a driveway and parking area.

At the opening dedication ceremony, it seemed that everyone came, including Minister Phumaphi and other government officials, US Ambassador John Lange, and the African regional head of UNAIDS. Mpule Kwelegobe, a former Miss Botswana who was now Miss Universe, also flew in from her world tour to participate. Mpule had become a vocal advocate for AIDS action, even convincing her successor, Miss India, to do the same. The band played, a chorus group sang, dancers danced, and President Mogae and I gave speeches. His was better than mine.

President Mogae repeated his pledge, which I had first heard him make more than a year before, that he would "never give a speech anywhere about anything without commenting on the scourge of HIV/AIDS." While Elizabeth and I were living in Botswana, we received numerous invitations to both private and government dinners and celebrations. The dinners were usually beef, to emphasize the growing local industry of grassfed beef, and President Mogae would speak. I remember one talk at the annual

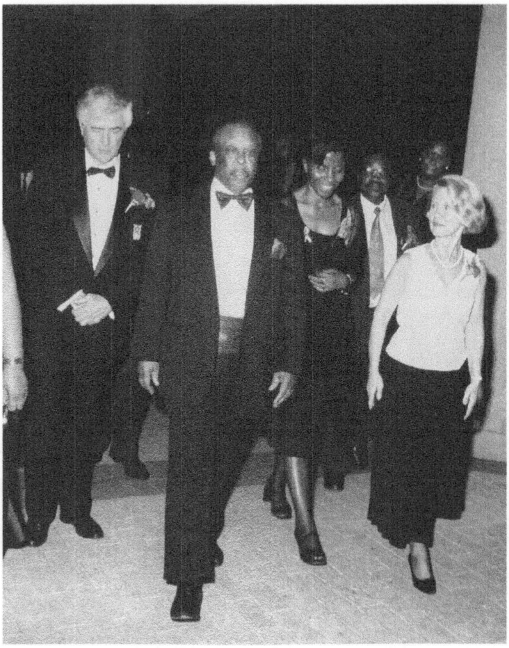

Figure 26.2: Max Essex, President Mogae, Minister Joy Phumaphi, Elizabeth Essex

agricultural fair where he spoke about the economic benefits of growing vegetables rather than importing them from South Africa. In the middle of the speech, he said, "Now I want to talk about AIDS." He did indeed follow that practice whenever I heard him speak, whether to a business group or to the police academy.

Now that we had a good functioning lab and funding from diverse sources like Merck, Bristol Myers Squibb, the US NIH, the Oak Foundation, and private donors, we wanted to move on to conducting trials. Having learned about the importance of community advisory boards for conducting AIDS trials in the United States, we sought to establish such an advisory committee in Botswana. It included representatives from the University of Botswana, the clergy, the business community, and the House of Chiefs. When I moved to Botswana, I also managed to bring three outstanding

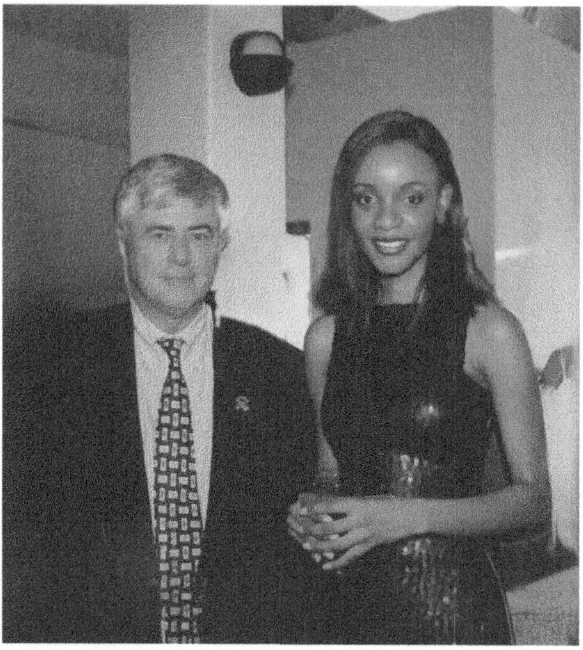

Figure 26.3: Max Essex, Mpule Kwelagobe

young women from our Boston group. One was Molly Pretorius Holme, an epidemiologist who had just married a South African tennis pro, Carel Pretorius, and welcomed the opportunity to be close enough to South Africa to get to know his family. The second was Tonya Villafana. Tonya was a native of Trinidad who had a public health degree from Harvard and a PhD in immunology from Cornell. She was an ideal person to head our vaccine section. She would later marry Ibou Thior, our first resident director of the Botswana Harvard Partnership (BHP). The third was Michelle Schaan, who had been in Botswana as a Peace Corps volunteer and knew the country well. Michelle would later earn a PhD, join the US Foreign Service, and get assigned to Ukraine during the Russian war.

With the goal of initiating vaccine trials, Tonya Villafana and I worked with two community representatives to raise awareness

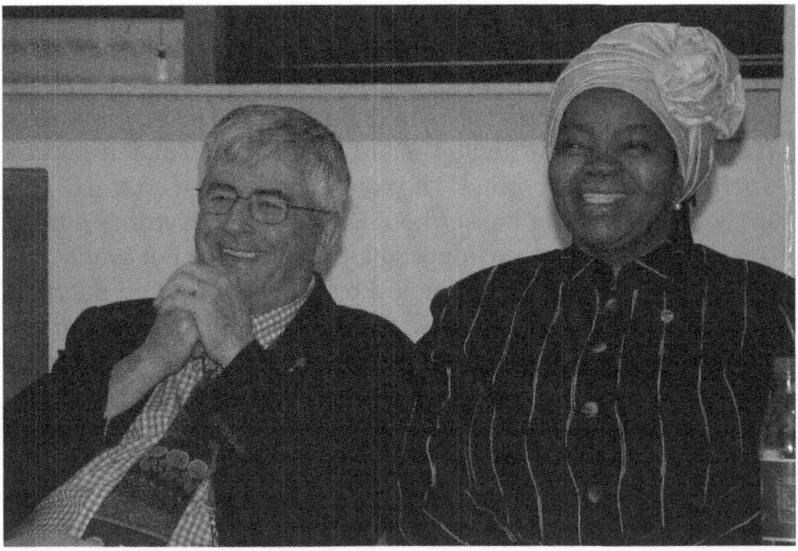

Figure 26.4: Max Essex, Sheila Tlou
Photo by Dave Cliff.

about the need for vaccine trials. Dr. Sheila Tlou was a PhD nurse and professor at the University of Botswana, where her husband Tom was a previous president and the leading historian on the history of the country. Sheila knew everyone, and everyone seemed to love her. She once took me to a working meeting of the Ntlo ya Dikgosi, or the meeting of the House of Chiefs, a group of about 20 Tswana tribal leaders who meet periodically to advise the Parliament about tribal rules and customs. Sheila spoke about the importance of participating as volunteers in vaccine trials. She was animated, but she spoke rapidly in Setswana, so I couldn't follow much of what she said. But I did understand her concluding statements when she asked, "How many of you chiefs would volunteer to be in a vaccine trial?" All raised their hands. And then we all clapped. Sheila, who had played the character of Mma Ramotswe for a local production of *The No. 1 Ladies' Detective Agency*, had endless charm. Later, she would also serve a term as minister of health.

Reverend Rupert Hambira was another person from the community who worked hard to help us begin clinical research trials. Rupert was president of the Council of Churches in Botswana. He was proud of his faith but also tired of officiating at the funerals of AIDS patients. Rupert invited me to speak about AIDS trials at a church service in Gaborone. The congregation seemed huge, perhaps 300 or 400. After the sermon, Rupert introduced me, stating that I would explain how important it was that the Botswana people participate in the trials. I gave a brief overview of all the trials we hoped to commence – vaccines, AIDS treatment, and mother/infant trials to prevent infant infections. People listened, but I couldn't tell how much they understood. I asked for questions. An elderly woman seated in the third row got up, came to the front of the room, and hugged me. It was Lady Masire, the wife of the former president. She spoke softly, but said, "I know this man. We can trust him. He is our friend." It almost brought me to tears. The congregation broke into applause.

Back in Boston, our lab group was working diligently to design a vaccine. Drs. Tun-Hou Lee and Vlad Novitsky were analyzing the outer surface of the gp120 molecule of the subtype C HIV to see which pieces of the protein would be most likely to stimulate the best antibodies and cellular immune responses.[158,159] Dr. Yichen Lu was designing a vaccine delivery system that we hoped would make the viral pieces even more immunogenic.[160] In the time period of 1998–2003, vaccine research represented the largest fraction of our lab research. We began vaccine trials in Botswana with two different designs. We determined that the experimental vaccines were safe but insufficiently immunogenic to stimulate a level of immunity that we thought would be required to protect against infection. As time went on, other research groups were designing and testing their own experimental HIV vaccines, but none showed promise. After investing so much time and resources on a vaccine, we were saddened, but soon we were uplifted by the new research opportunities for treatment and prevention with antiretroviral drugs (see chapter 17).

While on sabbatical in Botswana, I turned down most of the invitations I received to give talks, unless they were nearby in

Africa. On one occasion, Minister Joy Phumaphi called to ask if I could fill in for her to give a talk on AIDS, as she couldn't get back on time from a World Bank meeting in Europe. Joy was a friend who had helped me enormously, so I said of course I would. The talk was to be to a southern African convention of accountants at the Gaborone Sun Hotel. My host told a few of his accountant jokes and introduced me as the after-dinner speaker. I apologized for Minister Phumaphi and her travel problems, and then did my best to tell them about HIV/AIDS. At the end of my talk, the chairman had a photo-op where he presented me with a gift. It was a large silver knife for carving roasted meat, in a polished wooden box. On the box was a metal plaque that said "presented to Honorable Minister Joy Phumpahi" with the date. When I saw Joy about a week later, she asked me how the talk went. I said it was fine, and I have a gift for you that they left with me. She said, "No, no, you must keep it, you did the talk." I had visions of being stopped at airport security carrying a weapon engraved with the name of someone else. I then stopped by Joy's office at a time when I knew she was out and left the box.

When I was back in Boston, I had a visit from two young physicians, Shahin Lockman and Roger Shapiro. They said they wanted to work with me in Botswana. This seemed like a "wish come true." They had recently finished clinical training and certification in infectious diseases at the Harvard hospitals and had extra degrees in epidemiology. Both had previously lived in Africa, working for the US Centers for Disease Control and Prevention (CDC). I signed them on immediately, and they soon moved to Molepolole, Botswana, to help initiate our clinical trials to try to block transmission of HIV from infected pregnant women to their infants. As opposed to our attempts to make a vaccine, our research program to prevent infant infections has been immensely successful. After about 25 years as head of the Botswana program, I'd be retired. The program is still flourishing under the direction of Roger and Shahin in Boston, and Joe Makhema and Gaerolwe Masheto in Gaborone.

Our studies with maternal transmission of HIV from pregnant women to their infants had begun in Congo and continued in Tanzania and Thailand. Now we planned a massive expansion to include large trials in Botswana. In Congo, from studies done with Drs. Marc and Sophie Lallemant, we learned that certain immune correlates in the mother were predictive of neonatal transmission of HIV.[132] In Tanzania, our research with Drs. Wafaie Fawzi and Saidi Kapiga showed that different subtypes of HIV had preferential times for transmission.[161] Of particular relevance for Botswana, Dr. Boris Renjifo and our Boston lab found that HIV-1C was transmitted effectively from the mother at different stages of *in utero* development and delivery, as well as breastfeeding.[162,163] While our mother/infant trials in Thailand illustrated the ethical importance of conducting equivalence rather than placebo trials, they did not resolve the issue of what to do about infant infections that occurred as a result of breastfeeding.[137]

In most of the Global South, and especially Africa, the importance of breastfeeding has long been established as the best way to minimize infant deaths. Our challenge was to design trials for HIV-infected pregnant women so that their infected infants would be protected from HIV but also breastfed, so they'd also be protected from deaths due to pneumonias and diarrheal diseases. It had already been shown by others that formula feeding didn't work well in Africa. This was partly because of unclean infant formula and/or non-sterile feeding bottles but also because mother's milk provided protective antibodies to routine infant diseases, even if the mothers were HIV positive.

Dr. Steve Lagakos, a biostatistician friend at Harvard who had designed many drug trials, came up with a trial design for us that would allow us to test measures for both the *in utero* and the breastfeeding phases of infant infection at the same time. It was called a 2x2 factorial design. One of the problems we anticipated was enrolling the large number of HIV-positive pregnant women in the trial, about 1,200, to achieve statistical significance. More than one-third of pregnant women were HIV positive in Botswana, but birth rates were also declining. We succeeded, but only by setting up clinical trial teams in Mochudi, Molepolole, and Lobatse in addition to our home base at the BHP in Gaborone. Our experimental conclusion was marvelously gratifying. We found that breastfeeding could be done quite safely by HIV-positive mothers with appropriate drug prophylaxis. While infant HIV infections were not totally eliminated, their reduction was more than enough to offset infant deaths.[78] This was a huge first step that led to later studies by ourselves and others to show that drug treatment could be a tremendously important way to prevent HIV transmission in adults.[164,165]

By about 2004, BHP had expanded exponentially, with 330 employees in Botswana. More than 30 were physicians or PhD scientists. It was one of the most active sites for HIV/AIDS trials in the world. At Harvard, Dean Barry Bloom brought together a group of 25 current and prospective donors to travel to Africa to visit the project. Some were old friends, like Kate Sedgwick, Julie and Bayard Henry, and B Wu and Eric Larson. They visited the lab, the trial sites, and some of the local leaders. President Mogae graciously hosted a dinner for the entire group, including the leaders of our research team.

I had never considered myself to be very effective at fundraising or "development." I usually had the great fortune that others, like Michael Voligny and Kris Laping at Harvard, and especially Deeda Blair, were willing to do the asking. But I learned an important lesson during the 2004 visit of Dean Bloom with the Harvard visitors. Each day of the visit, I or another senior researcher gave a summary of what the visitors might expect to learn about the research. They would then travel an hour or so to Mochudi or Molepolole to visit the research clinics. One group met with HIV-positive mothers who had participated in the projects. Several of the mothers spoke, exuberantly saying things like, "My one-year-old boy here is healthy and HIV negative because of the research done by the Harvard doctors." That night, Susan Curren, a donor from the Boston area with connections to Harvard, said, "You know Max, you'd probably get more donations if you spoke less and let those mothers speak more." I hope I learned that lesson.

chapter twenty-seven

Treatment as Prevention and 90–90–90

As we expanded our program at the Botswana Harvard Partnership (BHP), it was becoming clear that antiretroviral (ARV) drugs had immense potential. The use of these drugs for AIDS patients in the United States, where they were often designated as HAART therapy, totally changed the face of AIDS. What was formerly a death sentence could now be survived, and with a reasonably good quality of life. It was almost analogous to the treatment of such disorders as diabetes and hypertension. As with drug therapy for the latter conditions, ARV for HIV/AIDS wasn't a cure, just a very effective way to stop disease progression. For some patients and populations, drug resistance would present new problems, but even these problems would soon be dealt with through the use of drug combinations. Consistent progress in ARV drug development and innovations for slow drug release would soon minimize relapses and side effects.

In the early 2000s, the lack of access to HAART in the Global South was a great concern. Soon after Jeff Sachs brought a group of us together at Harvard to campaign for AIDS drugs in third world countries, UNAIDS began lobbying for their "3 by 5" program – HAART treatment of 3 million African AIDS patients by 2005. The Harvard School of Public Health also had a new focus group on health disparities. So at the Harvard AIDS Institute (HAI) and BHP, we decided to learn all we could to make better use of the new wonder drugs where it mattered most.

President Mogae again demonstrated leadership, bringing us together to see what could be done with drugs in Botswana.

It was already clear that the country had been willing to invest in health care. Botswana had more financial capacity than most African countries. The small population was also an important feature that might be used to their advantage. As we negotiated with big pharma organizations like Merck or Bristol Myers Squibb for research drugs, it became clear that the companies were fearful of potential liability. The major concern drug companies have with new drugs in the United States is potential legal recourse for damages if the drugs cause harm. For drug trials in the developing world, companies have additional concerns. One is accusations that local people might be used as "guinea pigs," lacking access to adequate information to weigh risks versus benefits. This could cause serious reputational damage to pharmaceutical companies who test drugs in populations that do not have the financial capacity to purchase the drugs if they prove beneficial. If a company would feel obligated to later provide drugs for free or at reduced cost, it would be easier to do so in Botswana, with a population just above 2 million, than in a country like Nigeria, with a population of 200 million.

By now, many of the ARV drugs had been extensively tested in the United States and Europe. This meant that the specific drug-resistance mutations were well characterized for the virus of the West, HIV-1B. Yet none of these drug-resistance patterns had been elucidated for HIV-1C, the predominant virus for the world and the HIV that caused almost all of the infections in Botswana and the rest of southern Africa.

Our lab had determined the genetic codes of a large number of viruses from Botswana,[166] so we already could compare gene sites where mutations might be expected based on the published data for HIV-1B. At this point, very few people had been treated with ARV in Botswana, and we wanted to learn as much as possible before introducing the drugs to a large number of AIDS patients. I turned to an old friend at McGill University in Montreal, Dr. Mark Wainberg. Mark had discovered one of the main AIDS drugs. He had also devised some laboratory-based tests to select for drug-resistant HIV mutants without the need to wait for the disease-associated results of drug resistance in AIDS patients.

Mark invited me to give a lecture at McGill, and we made a plan to rapidly unravel the profile of drug resistance for the new virus as soon as possible.

While Mark studied our data for HIV-1C gene sequences as determined by Vlad Novitsky in my group, he'd also "drive" viral resistance to some key drugs in his lab cultures. This rapidly revealed some important new information about new drug-resistance mutations.[122] At the same time, Mark also sent one of his key deputies, Dr. Florence Doualla-Bell, to our lab in Botswana to teach us the techniques and to look at samples from local patients. Florence then worked with Drs. Simani Gaseitsiwe and Thumbi Ndung'u in the BHP lab to look at the first group of patients who were treated with ARV in Botswana. They, too, found some differences for HIV-1C that would help inform decisions about which ARV drugs might be most useful in Botswana.[167]

We soon began several new projects for ARV/HAART treatment of AIDS patients in Botswana. One was the KITSO program developed by Ric Marlink, our HAI executive director and a professor of public health from our department in Boston.[168] KITSO was a program developed to educate all physicians, nurses, and other health personnel in Botswana, about 40,000, so they could incorporate ARV into the treatment of AIDS patients and other HIV-infected persons such as pregnant women. The program was implemented by Christine Bussmann, an education specialist from Germany. Christine and her physician husband, Hermann, joined the BHP after many years of service at Deborah Retief Hospital in Mochudi, a town near Gaborone. Hermann would also help lead our clinical trials in HIV/AIDS patients.

Two more physicians, Drs. William and Carolyn Wester, also joined our team at BHP at just the time when we needed them. I first met Bill and Carolyn in a bar in Phnom Penh, Cambodia. The HOPE Foundation had asked me to help with a program they were developing there, and the Westers were there for the same reason. I enticed them to come to Botswana. They stayed for about 10 years, raising their three children in Gaborone. Bill, an infectious disease specialist, helped organize the adult treatment trials. Carolyn, an obstetrician and gynecologist, helped with our mother/infant trials.

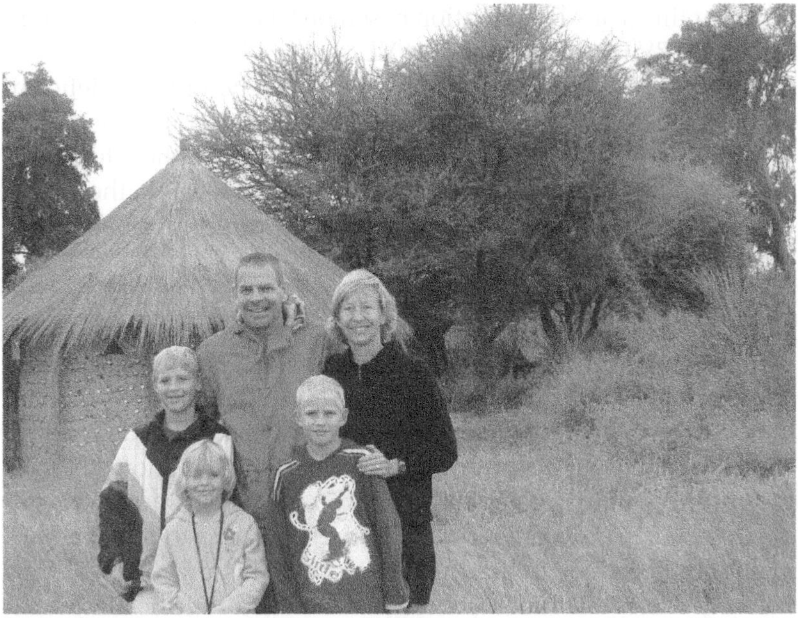

Figure 27.1: C. Wester, Maddie Wester, Bill Wester, Jimmy Wester, Carolyn Wester

When AIDS patients were first evaluated, their clinical stage of disease progression was based on the blood levels of a subset of lymphocytes called the CD4 cells. With normal levels at 600–1200, ARV treatment in the early days would only be initiated when the CD4 levels would get down to 300–400. It was thought that beginning ARV drugs earlier might also result in earlier drug resistance, resulting in a lack of effective drugs when they might be most needed. On the other hand, some thought that if ARVs were not used until the patient had deteriorated to 200 CD4 cells or below, it might be too late to save the life of the patient. Later, another blood test, viral load (VL), also became readily available. The VL was a better tool for predicting drug resistance and, along with CD4, a big help for estimating clinical prognosis of AIDS. We designed trials to look at all these parameters: different combinations of drugs, different times of ARV initiation based on CD4 levels, and different times of ARV initiation based on VL.

For the first group of about 600 severely immunodeficient patients treated in Botswana, the results were gratifying.[169] Following treatment, death rates were low, CD4 lymphocyte counts recovered, and VL levels were greatly reduced. Overall, the results were as good as, or better than, those reported for comparable groups of patients in the United States.

At about the same time, we noticed a potential problem with one of the ARV drugs, nevirapine, which was commonly used for prevention of mother-to-infant transmission. Nevirapine (NVP) was particularly helpful in situations where HIV-positive pregnant mothers did not get medical assistance until just before delivery. In some cases, the expectant mother would not even know she was HIV positive until delivery. When faced with such situations, single doses of NVP to the mother during labor and to the newborn infant could reduce infant infection rates. This practice was particularly useful in countries where women had little health care. It was also very inexpensive. However, a study organized by Shahin Lockman of our group also showed that this use of the drug could cause serious problems for ARV treatment of the mother. Namely, if mothers received the "birth NVP" for HIV prophylaxis of the infant, the mother would be much more likely to show drug resistance to NVP if she were given the same drug for her own health within the next 6 months.[170] And either NVP or the very closely related drug efavirenz, which had cross-reactive drug resistance, was usually a drug of choice for AIDS treatment at that time.

During this time period, I was also teaching a second-semester class to Harvard undergraduates. Their intelligence was readily apparent, as was their comprehension of HIV/AIDS. Many students inquired about the possibility of spending time in our lab, either in Boston or in Botswana. Working with Harvard college officials, we established a "semester abroad" program in Botswana. Designed for science-based pre-med undergraduates, we selected three young women for the first year in 2007. They took classes in Setswana, the native language, and African history at the University of Botswana, lived in dormitory rooms there, and

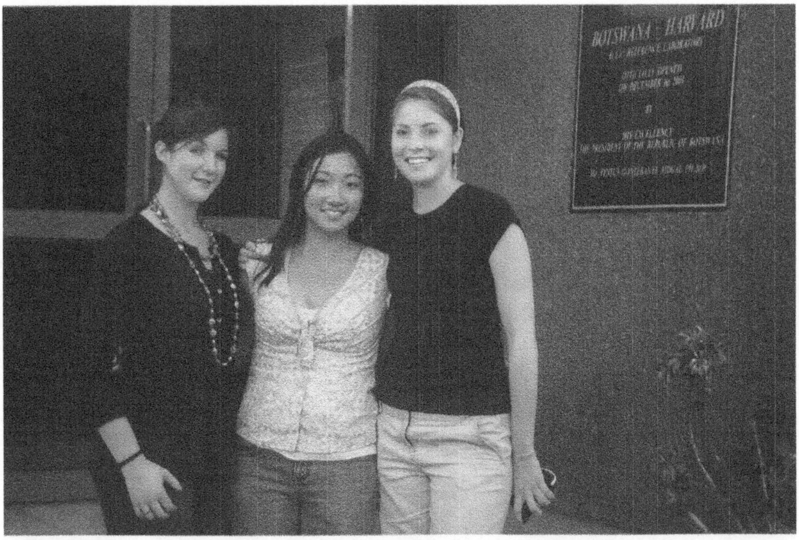

Figure 27.2: Lisa Flannery, Amy Wu, Jamie Greenwald

conducted a small research project in our BHP lab. For this, they would receive full credit for a semester at Harvard. The first three students selected for the program – Amy Wu, Jamie Greenwald, and Lisa Flannery – were superb. They seemed to love the experience and mentioned that it had a profound effect on their future careers.

Elizabeth and I also believed that our children and grandchildren should experience Africa. When they were teenagers, our daughters Holly and Carrie would spend time with us on safaris in Kenya and Tanzania. We took each of our grandchildren – Colin, Camille, Natalie, Anna, and Claire – to Botswana when they were eight. After he finished high school, Colin would go back to Mochudi for a time to teach sports in a school for disadvantaged children. Natalie would go to Ghana as a teacher's assistant during a gap year before beginning college at William and Mary.

Some of our most rewarding research results were from our trials to prevent mother/infant transmission of HIV in both Botswana and Thailand. If used correctly, we found that ARV could reduce

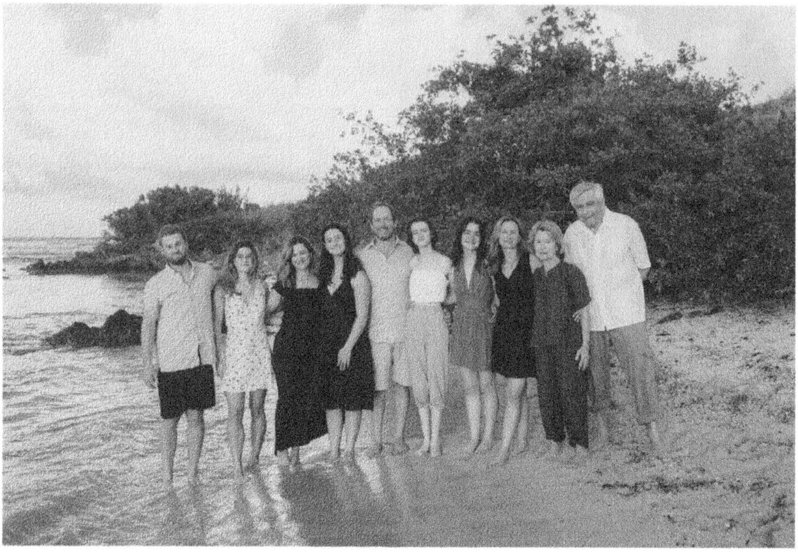

Figure 27.3: Max and Elizabeth Essex (right), with children and grandchildren

infant infections by at least 90%. This was a higher efficacy rate than we see with most vaccines. It led us to the obvious question about how effective ARV might be to prevent sexual transmission between adults. One of the most direct ways to evaluate this was by determining whether HIV-infected adults who were on ARV treatment were still able to transmit to their uninfected partners.

For the first trial, we collaborated with Dr. Mike Cohen, a friend at the University of North Carolina, who brought together research colleagues from eight different sites, mostly in Africa. The experimental design compared "discordant couples," where one sex partner in each pair was HIV infected and the partner was not infected. For ethical reasons, and equipoise, all HIV-infected partners were given ARV, but some were given the drugs later than others. Statistical analysis showed that 96% of the infections happened in couples where the infected partner did not take ARV for a greater period of sexual exposure.[171] A genetic analysis of HIV sequences done by a former student of mine, Dr. Andrew Redd, confirmed that the new infections had come from the infected partner in the trial rather than from a sexual partner from outside the relationship.

While this was going on, we also got a grant from the US National Institutes of Health (NIH) to test the concept of "treatment as prevention," or TasP, in a large village population. We selected Mochudi, which had a population of about 40,000 and was less than an hour from BHP in Gaborone. Our approach, which was new, was to mobilize the ARV TasP based on VL rather than CD4 lymphocyte levels or clinical disease. We did this because we found that people infected in southern Africa with HIV-1C often demonstrated a sustained high VL, more so than had been reported for other viral subtypes like HIV-1B.[172] This seemed important because higher VL was clearly associated with higher rates of transmission. Thus, we could focus our ARV-mediated TasP on a subset of HIV-infected people we might think of as "hypertransmitters." Another aspect of our approach was to use the genetic sequences from new HIV infections in Mochudi to match them to an infectious "source person" based on phylogenetic matching of the viruses.[173]

The study in Mochudi showed that this new approach was possible but also that we'd need a larger population of people to achieve statistical significance. Also, it seemed that the use of smaller villages that were more isolated than Mochudi might increase our sensitivity for detecting transmission networks. This led us to a huge undertaking called the Botswana Combination Prevention Project (BCPP), or Ya Tsie in the Setswana language. "Ya tsie" means "teamwork is better than individual effort."

To design Ya Tsie, I worked closely with Dr. Victor DeGruttola, the chair of the biostatistics department at Harvard. The plan we devised was based on community randomization. We would select 30 villages that were as isolated as possible to minimize the proportion of HIV infections that originate outside the village for any new cases of HIV infection. The villages would be located throughout the country, though most of the population of Botswana is based in the eastern and southeastern parts of the country. Only villages that had from 3,000 to 12,000 people would be included. The 30 villages would be categorized as "pairs," based on similarities in size, geographical location, and other demographic criteria. The pairs would each be randomized such that one village in each pair would receive the special TasP VL intervention. Citizens of all 30 villages would receive the national standards for HIV prevention and treatment, as well as extra prevention interventions like voluntary male circumcision, condoms, and intensified health care. The villages selected had a total population of adults from about 74,000 households. We estimated that it would take about 3 years to complete the study after enrollment. Our design would include HIV tests for all who were willing to participate but also HIV viral genetic linkage mapping of all available samples done by Vlad Novitsky in my lab.

We estimated that the entire Ya Tsie would cost at least $35 million, maybe more. We presented the proposal to the Gates Foundation. They were interested but reluctant to spend that much money on a single project. We then submitted the same proposal to the US government. They approved the plan, with the caveat that the US Centers for Disease Control and Prevention (CDC) could also be involved. This created the usual bureaucratic delays often associated with governmental activities but also increased the budget to about $70 million. The leader of the CDC section that had the responsibility was Dr. Debi Birx, whom I knew. As mentioned before, Birx would later become the White House point person for COVID.[139]

The TasP project was ultimately successful. The expanded HIV testing and treatment strategy resulted in a lower rate of new HIV infections, especially within those villages that received the most ARV.[164,165,174] Subsequent studies by Dr. Lerato Magosi, a Motswana postdoctoral fellow at Harvard, extended the study using viral genetics to link transmissions.[175] As expected, transmissions into intervention communities from control communities were more common than the reverse.

These results were only possible because of the ingenuity shown by our fellow researchers at BHP in Gaborone under the leadership of Dr. Makhema. His deputy, Dr. Mompati Mmalane, was the "front man" who first went to each village to educate and negotiate with tribal leaders. He was one of the few local Botswana leaders who achieved great success in medicine even before the existence of a medical school in the country. From a small rural village origin and college in Botswana, he was granted a scholarship to study medicine at the University of Tübingen. With no background in German, he became fluent in 6 months.

Another outstanding clinical research physician who contributed immensely to these studies is Dr. Tendani Gaolathe. In addition to her key role in the Ya Tsie program, Tendani also led a study evaluation of the national program of ARV treatment.

In 2015, UNAIDS began to push an evaluation strategy that was based on TasP called 90–90–90. The UN goals for each country were that 90% of HIV-positive people should know they are infected based on extensive testing; 90% of those who are HIV positive based on this testing should be on ARV drug therapy; and 90% of those on ARV therapy should have low VL based on testing. The target for reaching the goals was to be 2020. If these goals were met, UNAIDS estimated that the HIV pandemic would be over by 2030, at least in epidemic form.[176] In a publication in *Lancet*, Tendani represented many of us with an analysis showing that Botswana had almost reached that goal by 2016.[174] Botswana was the first country in Africa to meet this 90–90–90 goal and one of the first in the world to do so. In fact, we estimated that the country had reached 95–95–95 before 2020.[165] This has to be considered a major achievement, especially for President Mogae and for the importance of good governmental policy for public health.

Because of the amazing accomplishments and competence of my former students and colleagues, I am no longer needed in Botswana. Elizabeth and I will still enjoy traveling to see old friends and to experience the magical charm of Africa.

For a holiday treat, we decided to go to Madagascar, the large island country off the coast of southeast Africa. Our goal was to find lemurs, the primitive species of monkeys that are native to that country. We landed in Antananarivo and drove to the forests of the north. We hired a local guide to lead us in the dense forest. After an hour or so, he told us to stay in one spot, saying he would go off alone to find lemurs. I found myself wondering what we would do if he failed to return. We seemed to be miles from people or even any clear paths. He did come back and led us deeper into the forest where he had spotted a band of lemurs. We went to the site and offered the animals pieces of mango. They were wild but seemingly unafraid, sitting on our shoulders as long as we had food to give them. It reminded me of the Galapagos Islands where the animals and birds lack sufficient evolutionary experience with the human species to be afraid.

We also accepted a special offer to visit Lion Camp, a site in the Okavango Delta where a husband-and-wife team of naturalists from South Africa studies lions. The Okavango Delta is unique, the largest delta in the world. It is filled by the Okavango River, which becomes swollen by the seasonal rains in Angola. Our friend Dr. Steve O'Brien, the US geneticist, has a permanent tent at the compound, which he let us use. We were there when the delta was at the peak rate of filling, with water pouring onto the Kalahari Desert. As the water covers the sand, hordes of insects are washed out of their holes. A wave of frogs, snakes, and small birds then appear to eat the insects, just ahead of another wave of large birds and mammals that eat the reptiles. Herds of antelope come to drink at the flooded pans, and they are followed by the lions.

chapter twenty-eight

Pandemic Politics

During the last 40 years, two major pandemics have occurred. For the first, HIV/AIDS, the best estimates are that 40 million people died and another 40–50 million are still infected.[177] For the second, COVID, the estimates are that 6–8 million people have died and almost a billion have been infected. Medical research that produced drugs and vaccines for these infections saved hundreds of millions more from infection and/or death. Combinations of new drugs for HIV/AIDS saved the lives of infected people and made them non-contagious so that they don't spread HIV to others.[165] Rapidly developed vaccines for COVID prevented serious infections and made minimally infected people non-infectious to others.[178] The vaccines could eliminate COVID epidemics if most adults got vaccinated. Current attitudes toward vaccines and other public health measures made it unlikely that this would happen. Drugs for COVID also saved many lives and made many COVID-infected people less likely to infect others.

Both pandemics originated as viral zoonoses, new to the human species (see chapters 15 and 16). The first began from apes in Africa, the second from bats in China. We should expect more new epidemics and more of these epidemics to become pandemics. Viruses evolve much faster than people can counter with an evolutionary response against them. Pigs, ducks, camels, civets, and other species serve as amplifiers to fast-forward the transfer to humans of viral pathogens like flu and COVID. Urbanization and air travel have also exacerbated the epidemics. Climate change and the associated natural disasters could play an even larger role for the spread of infections in the future.

Perhaps the greatest success story for public health was the worldwide eradication of smallpox, which happened almost 50 years ago. This project was successful for two major reasons. The first was the nature of the viral disease itself. All people who get infected readily reveal their condition as a skin rash that is almost pathognomonic – distinctive for the disease. An effective vaccine was readily available. As soon as cases were identified, all the people in the surrounding community could be vaccinated to block the possibility that the infection would be transmitted. Teams of physicians and public health officials were dispatched to all corners of the globe by the World Health Organization. They were armed with the vaccine provided jointly by the United States and the Soviet Union. The second reason the eradication was successful was international cooperation and political will. It would be farfetched to imagine such success in our current political environment.

As a virologist and an infectious disease researcher, I am often asked my opinion on whether we will have another pandemic like HIV/AIDS or COVID. My answer is yes. The more difficult questions relate to what type of virus it might be, how it might start, and how it might be transmitted. The most difficult question to answer is how we could stop it. Lassa, Ebola, and mpox (formerly called monkey pox) are scary viruses that periodically enter the human population as zoonoses, sometimes causing small epidemics, especially in Africa. But these viruses cause distinctive signs and symptoms, so cases can be rapidly identified and kept away from transmission chains. For Ebola and mpox, vaccines already exist.

HIV and the COVID virus caused epidemics or pandemics because massive transmission occurred before we realized an epidemic was present. With HIV, individuals spread the virus for years before they realized they had a disease. With COVID, the signs and symptoms for most were the same as the signs and symptoms of other infectious respiratory viruses. COVID, flu, and respiratory syncytial virus all have RNA genomes, which encourages the generation of mutant variants. Some of the mutants will be more transmissible. Some will be more lethal. We now have techniques for rapidly sequencing the genomes of many viruses at once from the body fluids of patients with respiratory diseases and even from healthy carriers. This can and should be done more often on representative populations throughout the world. We also have rapid diagnostic tests that can be used in a clinic or at home.

After the worldwide eradication of smallpox, a committee was established to recommend action on the destruction of existing laboratory stocks of the virus.[179] I was on the committee, representing the National Academy of Medicine. We were told that only two stocks of viable smallpox virus were maintained in the world in freezers, one at the US Centers for Disease Control and Prevention in Atlanta and one in Moscow. One side of the debate was that these two viral stocks should be eliminated to avoid possible escape of the virus from the laboratories. The other side, which I was aligned with, felt that the virus stocks should be maintained to allow new research in case it might be needed in the future. Some of us speculated that additional samples of smallpox virus might already exist, unbeknownst to the authorities. If such a virus were released, whether inadvertently or deliberately, perhaps as a bioweapon, it would be important to have the reference virus from Atlanta or Moscow to help design drugs and vaccines. My experience of unexpectedly finding the 1918 Alaskan feet with flu virus in my own lab freezer factored into my opinion (see chapter 4). It seems ironic that mpox itself is now causing a new, albeit limited, epidemic in our own population. Like HIV, mpox came from an animal reservoir in tropical Africa and is spread most efficiently by sexual contact. But unlike HIV, mpox outbreaks have usually been limited to a small number of people.

The infectious disease that was next on the list for worldwide eradication was polio. That goal is already 25 years behind the original target date, but it could happen. One of the last pockets of cases is in Afghanistan. The Taliban, however, seemed to be cooperating.[180] We might contrast that with the situation in Florida under Governor DeSantis, where his surgeon general is defying long-standing practices to control measles, like using the very effective childhood vaccines.[181] Outbreaks of this highly contagious virus have occurred recently in the state. For measles, which could have been eradicated years ago, we are now going backward.

Public health malpractice has become rampant. Unlike most practicing physicians, politicians need no license to practice or create public health policy. Uninformed charlatans simply declare themselves to be vaccine experts, ignore consensus health data, and recommend against constructive action.

A team of experts recently published an extensive analysis of the US government response to the COVID-19 pandemic.[182] Their conclusion was that the US response was little more than chaos, "a collective national incompetence in government. Despite having more capabilities than any other country, we had one of the least effective responses to the epidemic." One recent study reported that COVID mortality rates were 11% higher in states with Republican-controlled governments and 26% higher in areas where voters lean conservative.[183] Another study found that Republican counties had a 43% higher COVID mortality rate as compared to Democratic counties in Florida and Ohio.[103] The anti-vaccine movement is also gaining power in Republican statehouses.[184] Economists David Cutler and Lawrence Summers estimated that the COVID-19 epidemic cost the country $16 trillion in economic output, business failure, lost education, unemployment, and lost lives.[185] The creation of a national commission to organize for the next pandemic should seem like a dirt cheap investment in relation to cost-effectiveness. Under another Trump administration, things could get much worse.

Many of us have celebratory memories about the President's Emergency Plan for AIDS Relief (PEPFAR) created by President George W. Bush in 2003. PEPFAR saved tens of millions of lives by providing AIDS drugs to people in countries that were hit hardest by HIV/AIDS. Bush's presentation of the program fit an image he initially projected as a "Christian conservative" and a "compassionate conservative." The PEPFAR program did more than any other recent US action to win the hearts and minds of people in the Global South. Several of the countries designated for benefits were those that Trump called the "shithole countries" that should be avoided. I've worked in several of these countries and found the people to be kind, generous, and eager to cooperate, usually lacking the avarice and cynicism that is becoming more common in the United States.

Following authorization of the PEPFAR program by Congress, four groups were awarded competitive contracts to provide education and drugs for AIDS disease treatment and protection. The largest contract was to the Catholic Relief Organization, who partnered with the Institute of Human Virology at the University of Maryland for medical expertise. One of the four contracts was to my former student and then faculty colleague at Harvard, Dr. Phyllis Kanki. Phyllis mobilized large, impactful projects in Nigeria, Tanzania, and Botswana.

In 2019, I became the Lasker Professor Emeritus at Harvard. Friends and colleagues organized events for celebration both in Boston and in Botswana. President Mogae came to both events. A few months later, I broke my neck, fracturing three vertebrae while hiking on a rocky trail in Borderland State Park. My neurosurgeon said that most people who get these injuries don't survive. My recovery took months of immobilization, tube feeding, medications, and nursing by Elizabeth. In the end, I recovered.

My education began in a lower middle-class public school in a New England mill town. My father left school in the eighth grade to work in the local cotton mill. When I was in high school, a third or more of the boys worked in the same mill when they reached 16. Some of the boys in my class put in a 3–11 pm 40-hour workweek while they were still in school. To me, school seemed easy. We had little homework, perhaps to accommodate those who worked in full-time jobs.

Jesse Stone once said, "If you want to have an interesting life, hang around with people who are smarter than you are."[186] This seemed to work for me. I have been very fortunate to have spent most of my time doing that.

chapter twenty-nine

An Impending Public Health Disaster

It is inauguration day, January 20, 2025. Newly elected President Trump said he would be a dictator on day 1. About 8 hours after taking the oath of office, he signs an executive order for the United States to withdraw from the World Health Organization (WHO), a branch of the United Nations. The reason for doing so, he said, was because the UN "mishandled the response to the COVID-19 epidemic."

Based on national numbers for death and disease, many would argue that it was the United States that had badly botched the response to COVID-19. In April 2020, at the peak of COVID expansion, Trump spoke at a White House briefing about the epidemic. He challenged his health officials to investigate the possibility of injecting bleach or using very powerful ultraviolet light. Standing nearby, Dr. Deborah Birx, the White House coronavirus coordinator, seemed to cringe. "It was the craziest and most surreal moment I had ever witnessed in a presidential press conference," said Jonathan Karl, ABC's chief Washington correspondent.[187] Happening just months before the election of 2020, that episode set off a tsunami of criticism of the government for their handling of the epidemic.

By 2 years into the COVID epidemic, about 1 million Americans had died of the disease. After good vaccines were available, death rates were higher in Republicans for states where vaccine uptake rates were low, like Florida and Ohio. Deaths were more than 2.5 times higher in the 300 counties that were most pro-Trump as compared to the 300 most anti-Trump counties.[188] COVID would go on to cause an economic depression as steep as any in recent memory. Some estimated the cost to be as high as $15 trillion in the US.

The US withdrawal from the WHO could have grave consequences for the United States when the next epidemic occurs. We may lose access to data about where in the world the flu, COVID, Marburg, mpox, or Ebola virus is moving. This has obvious implications for protection of the homeland. But it should also be a major concern for the Department of Defense. US military bases exist in many parts of the world for strategic reasons. If an infectious disease strikes in a region with ongoing unrest, and we are unaware of it, our troops may be vulnerable and ineffective. They may also return from such places bringing new viruses and epidemics to the homeland.

By withdrawing from the WHO, we will also lose rapid access to case materials from new outbreaks. Such patient materials may be needed to make drugs and vaccines.

Frightening outbreaks of Marburg virus have recently occurred in Africa. Like some others, Marburg virus usually comes to human populations from bats. It is as deadly as Ebola, killing 20–80%. There is reason to believe we could make a good vaccine for Marburg, as one was already made for a strain of Ebola that caused a lethal outbreak in West Africa. But to do this, we would need rapid access to blood samples from the developing outbreak. This may be difficult if the local government distrusts US motives, and the United States is no longer involved with the WHO.

The United States, especially through the Centers for Disease Control and Prevention (CDC), has usually played an outsized role in shaping WHO policy and response to new epidemics. Those seats at the WHO table may well be filled by China.

The WHO was also condemned because it was working on a treaty to strengthen pandemic preparedness and set legally binding policies for member countries to share data rapidly. This proposed agreement was viewed by some as a threat to US national sovereignty. According to Larry Gostin, a professor of public health law at Georgetown University, this could "leave the CDC flying blind."[189]

Trump's nominee to be head of the Department of Health and Human Services (HHS) was Robert F. Kennedy Jr. RFK Jr. has the dubious title of head of the anti-vaxxers, a social movement that uses misinformation to discourage vaccinations. Vaccinations are, of course, our most important tool for preventing epidemics. Trump's first pick to head the CDC, our lead agency for preventing infectious diseases, was Dave Weldon. Weldon has also been a leading anti-vaxxer. After it became clear that the nomination of Weldon would be voted down by the Senate, Trump withdrew his nomination.

In his own Senate confirmation hearings, RFK Jr. stated that he wasn't against vaccines, though many don't believe him because of his previous statements. Kennedy emphasizes a libertarian position, stating that vaccination should be a personal choice. But when the personal choice results in rampant epidemics of highly transmissible viral diseases due to an absence of herd immunity, the burden of disease, death, and hospital costs are borne by the entire population.

The chairman of the committee charged with reviewing Kennedy's nomination was Senator Bill Cassidy of Louisiana. He sought to get reassurance from Kennedy that he would not interfere with the use of essential vaccines and that he would keep the important CDC Advisory Committee on Immunization Practices. After he was confirmed, RFK Jr. canceled the committee meeting that was scheduled to design the makeup of the next flu vaccine and canceled the federal contract that the government had awarded to make the vaccine. He soon fired all 17 members of the vaccine advisory committee. He replaced them with a smaller group that lacked vaccine experience but were known to be sympathetic to his anti-vax positions. Robert Malone, the co-chair of the new committee, said he considered the term "anti-vaxxer" to be high praise.[190] Kennedy also fired the Food and Drug Administration (FDA)'s top vaccine scientist.

RFK Jr. minimizes the importance of infectious diseases and thus the role of vaccines in disease prevention. He claimed that the CDC and the FDA were "a rubber stamp" or "sock puppets for industry."[191] He also claimed that he would bar National Institutes of Health (NIH) scientists from publishing in the most respected medical journals such as *The New England Journal of Medicine* and the *Journal of the American Medical Association* because they were supposedly controlled by the pharmaceutical companies.

Kennedy has also been a major party to a legal action against Merck concerning their vaccine against the viruses that cause cervical cancer. He and his fellow litigants claimed that Merck failed to warn consumers that the vaccine was only effective against "certain cancers." The vaccine, a breakthrough in medical research, protects against cervical and vaginal cancers and is now used throughout the world. It is recommended by the US CDC as a routine immunization for 11- or 12-year-olds. Available since 2006, more than 160 million doses have been used in the United States.

Kennedy further damaged the image of the United States in the world as he stated his recommendation that the United States stop contributing to Gavi, the global vaccine alliance. Gavi has helped vaccinate more than a billion children since the year 2000 and has reduced childhood deaths by as much as 50%.[192] Without consulting with experts, RFK Jr. also withdrew the CDC recommendation that pregnant women and children receive the COVID vaccine. This resulted in a suit filed by the leading public health organizations.[193] If infected and unvaccinated, pregnant women may be at higher risk for miscarriage and stillbirths. More recently, at the recommendation of RFK Jr., the US government has scaled back the number of vaccines recommended for children.[194]

At about the same time Kennedy began as the new secretary of health and human services, a new outbreak of measles was beginning in the United States. Almost all unvaccinated people get measles if exposed. Measles is the most contagious virus known to exist. About 90% of those who are exposed get infected unless they have been vaccinated. The virus is airborne, moving through pediatric populations like wildfire. As with most human viruses, measles originally came from animals, probably from rinderpest in cattle. Fortunately, a very effective vaccine is available for measles. It was made by a friend of mine, the late Maurice Hilleman. It has been estimated that this vaccine has prevented the deaths of at least 50 million children. The vaccine is exceptionally safe. This is salient because to stop an epidemic 95% or more of the population must be vaccinated. Before widespread vaccination, measles was the most common cause of blindness and hearing loss in children.

The new outbreak in the United States started in west Texas in early 2025. The spread was clearly associated with a downturn in childhood vaccination. By July, there were about 1,300 cases and 3 deaths, the highest level seen in 33 years. While about 95% of children must be vaccinated for herd immunity, mistrust about the measles, mumps, rubella (MMR) vaccine had greatly increased in the area. In one study, vaccination rates had fallen to 90% among Democrats and 68% among Republicans.[195] More than 2,000 cases of measles were reported in the United States during 2025, the highest number in more than 30 years.[196]

As it turned out, Kennedy had prior experience with a serious outbreak of measles in Samoa. The country of Samoa is in Polynesia. Most of the 200,000 residents live on its two large islands. In 2019, it had a major epidemic of measles that killed about 3% of the country's young children. The tragedy was preceded by a hospital accident in which a nurse mistakenly mixed two doses of measles vaccines with a toxic diluent. This initiated fear about the safety of the MMR vaccine, which had previously been used safely throughout the world for decades. Kennedy and his anti-vaxxers saw an opportunity to move in, which caused a major disaster. As chairman of Children's Health Defense, his anti-vaccine nonprofit organization, RFK Jr. visited Samoa and raised concerns about vaccination to the prime minister.

When the epidemic hit, childhood vaccination rates had fallen to about 30%. Other nearby islands that were not part of Samoa, where vaccination rates were above 95%, had no epidemic of measles. Yet Kennedy sent the Samoan prime minister a letter suggesting that the measles cases could have been due to vaccination. The director-general of Samoa's health ministry said that RFK Jr., if he becomes US secretary of HHS, may be directly responsible for killing thousands of children "by empowering the anti-vax movement, which would allow preventable infectious diseases to run rampant."[197] Josh Green, a physician who was governor of Hawaii, stated, "RFK Jr. had spread so much misinformation that the country [Samoa] stopped vaccinating, and that caused a tragic and fatal spread of measles."[198]

Kennedy has also indicated his intention to suspend research on infectious diseases for 8 years.

Soon after the inauguration, the NIH and other federal funding agencies like the CDC were told that they are prohibited from spending funds that have already been allocated. Research studies may be interrupted or terminated. Some, such as clinical research trials with human subjects, are very expensive, and they may go on for 3–6 years, involving hundreds or thousands of human volunteers. The minimum number of participants to be enrolled to obtain a meaningful result is calculated before the trial is initiated. The number is based on statistical powering projections designed to give confidence that any final result, whether it be drug or vaccine efficacy or toxicity, would not be due to random chance. With even limited interruptions in participant visits and data collection, the value of the entire trial may be at risk. Along with the commitments of trial participants, staff, and research scientists, the trials typically represent investments of tens or hundreds of millions of dollars that may be lost.

The anti-vax movement is older than RFK Jr., but it received a big boost through the Children's Health Defense fund he chaired. A chief strategy of both Kennedy and Children's Health Defense has been to question the safety of medicines, usually based on misinterpretation of the science or outright support of fraudulent studies. Couched in the language of "freedom to make your own health decisions," they have succeeded in scaring enough parents away from having their children vaccinated to deprive the entire population of the benefits of "herd immunity." If enough children remain unvaccinated, because of ignorance or fear, the entire population becomes vulnerable, eliminating the benefits of the public health process. It seems fair to say that if an organization like Children's Health Defense had been in place and effective 50–70 years ago, smallpox would not have been eradicated. This organization and RFK Jr. have contributed immensely to our failure to eliminate polio and measles.

During recent decades, the rates of diagnosed autism have increased dramatically. Diagnosis of autism often occurs at about the same time children first receive vaccines for diseases like measles, mumps, and rubella (MMR). Anti-vaxxers questioned whether either the vaccines themselves or the scheduling of multiple vaccines together caused autism. The role of thimerosal, which was used as a preservative for some vaccines, was also considered as a possible culprit. But the use of thimerosal in childhood vaccines was stopped decades ago, and new diagnoses of autism continue to rise.

Dr. Allen Frances, an eminent psychiatrist at Duke University, has a good explanation for why the rates of autism have increased dramatically in recent decades. He believes it is nothing more than an increase in diagnosis related to a reclassification to what is now called the autism spectrum disorder. Dr. Allen was chair of a task force charged with finding a new definition of autism for the *Diagnostic and Statistical Manual of Mental Disorders*.[199] The goal was to change the definition, previously restricted to very early onset symptoms, to include late onset behavioral problems. This was done in part to provide better health care and special services in schools.

RFK Jr. has also been associated with a fringe industry that exploited autism for profit. This included dubious measures for prevention and treatment. It has been reported that Kennedy earned about $2.5 million from one law firm for referring autism clients.[200]

A father-and-son team, Mark and David Geier, were among the leaders of this "autism for profit" industry. Mark Geier was a Maryland physician whose license was revoked over concerns about his false credentials and unconventional treatments for autism. He was an expert witness for more than 90 plaintiffs in vaccine injury suits. He also had eight clinics to treat autistic children, at about $5,000 per month per patient, with the drug Lupron, which acts by chemical castration.[201] For this, he lost his license. David Geier had no medical license or training and was disciplined in Maryland for practicing medicine without a license. He had also collaborated with his father to publish a paper about thimerosal as a cause of autism. The paper was soon retracted by the journal. In March 2025, Kennedy hired David Geier to conduct a new governmental study on whether vaccines cause autism.

In 1998, a paper was published claiming that the MMR vaccine was linked to a novel form of enterocolitis and autism.[202] It was soon obvious that the study was poorly designed, lacking controls. Even worse, investigators soon showed that the study was fraudulent.[203] It was retracted by the journal *The Lancet*, who originally published the paper, and the principal author, Andrew Wakefield, lost his medical license and was dismissed from his position. Many other studies were conducted. The US National Academy of Medicine, among others, concluded there was no association between MMR vaccines and autism. One study of more than half a million children in Denmark saw no association between autism and measles vaccinations. But the damage caused through faulty education of the public could not be easily corrected. Andrew Wakefield, like the Geiers, spent more than two decades publicly perpetuating dangerous misinformation about vaccines. They were assisted, if not led, by RFK Jr. as a conspiracist leader.

Much of the long-term damage done by anti-vaxxer Andrew Wakefield was unraveled by the award-winning British journalist Brian Deer in his book *The Doctor Who Fooled the World*.[203] It should be mandatory reading for RFK Jr. and other anti-vaxxers.

Some other journalists have done more harm than good. Edward Hooper published *The River*, proposing that AIDS originated from oral polio vaccines that were supposedly contaminated by vaccine virus grown in chimpanzee cells.[204] This was disproven by substantial evidence. *Rolling Stone* magazine published a similar story, blaming the origin of HIV/AIDS on oral polio vaccine virus grown on monkey kidney cells.[205] That polio vaccine was made by Drs. Albert Sabin and Hilary Koprowski. Hilary, whom I knew well, was responsible for the first human trial, which was conducted in Congo. He sued the author and *Rolling Stone*, and won. They published an apology.

Most pharmaceutical companies are uninterested in making vaccines, a type of product that is usually used only once or twice by consumers. By contrast, drugs are large market items. Those used for chronic diseases like hypertension, depression, or diabetes may be used daily for life, providing a much larger market. To encourage the making of vaccines, the government has sometimes had to offer major incentives in advance, as the Department of Defense frequently does for expensive weapons. For example,

Congress passed the Childhood Vaccine Injury Act to protect vaccine makers and ensure an adequate supply of vaccines. More recently, coronavirus vaccine makers were given large government contracts to respond rapidly to the needs of the epidemic.

The use of medical malpractice legal action is usually viewed as an appropriate response to the faulty application of medical services that results in bodily harm. Among the downsides are the expense of malpractice insurance. Ultimately borne by all of us as health-care consumers, the costs for specialties such as surgery and obstetrics may be hundreds of thousands of dollars per year for each physician. Legal measures for meaningful responses to public health malpractice are much harder to define and to mobilize. At the core of public health are the disciplines of epidemiology and biostatistics. Many, if not most, public health administrators lack expertise in these subjects.

Who might be defined as a practitioner of public health policy in most governmental systems? President Trump could probably not be sued for expressing an opinion that research should be done on injecting bleach for COVID infections. Could he be sued for nominating a director of HHS who is against vaccines? Kennedy could probably not be sued for encouraging the US NIH to divert research dollars to investigate whether vaccines cause autism, a topic that most believe is settled science. Could Kennedy and the government be sued if unvaccinated pregnant women get infected with COVID and suffer stillbirths? Perhaps. What about when unvaccinated children become blinded or die from measles after a parent was brainwashed against vaccines?

No good examples of public health malpractice suits against the government exist. The successful class action suit against the tobacco companies may give some precedent for process and standing, but it was not against a government. While it resulted in a more than $200 billion payout, it took three decades to resolve, and it still represents a tiny fraction of the costs of health care and lives lost due to tobacco-related illnesses.

Many experts believe that our next pandemic will be bird flu, some version of H5N1, and that it is "right around the corner." Most flu viruses are seen first in wild migrating waterfowl in Asia.

They move west, infecting animals like pigs and cattle along the way, and subsequently people. Genetic changes in the virus are common, resulting both from mutations and by reassortment when two different types of viruses infect the same individual host cell. A "hybrid virus" then emerges having some of the characteristics of both parental strains. The new virus may be easier to transmit, or more lethal, or both. Many virologists are wondering why this hasn't happened already since some bird and livestock populations already seem saturated with H5N1. Scientists and public health experts are urging expanded surveillance of both human and animal populations. Some argue that the recent cancellation of an annual flu vaccine contract may be the most serious mistake of all the recent blunders by Kennedy.[206]

But what if our next pandemic is something worse than flu – harder to predict and harder to contain? This is the situation that faced us with our last two epidemics. Forty-five years ago, when HIV/AIDS began, no experts predicted the arrival of a new sexually transmitted virus that would attack our immune system. It was a virus type not known to exist in humans, and a sexual way of spreading that left epidemiologists, and everyone else, confused about how to respond until it was too late. Forty million people died before it could be controlled.

Our next pandemic surfaced in 2019, and it also found us unprepared. In retrospect, we should have been expecting it – we had had warnings through smaller COVID epidemics in Hong Kong in 2003 and in the Middle East in 2012. COVID-19 still took us by surprise, overwhelming government public health agencies, medical services, social conventions, and global health networks.

Logic would suggest we should plan for a new "unexpected" type of pandemic within the next 10–20 years. What if our next pandemic is caused by a new virus that is airborne, like measles, but different, like HIV, so that we have no precedent for finding a solution? Could it come again from Asia or Africa, or perhaps even from encroachments on the Amazon rainforest where we have no knowledge of viruses harbored by the indigenous fauna?

To reduce major destruction by the next pandemic, we need better surveillance through governmental agencies and international cooperation, and more research on virus evolution and infectious diseases. We also need a plan for societal implementation of prevention and treatment when faced with the reality of the situation.

Suspension of research, destruction of public health agencies, hostility toward international collaboration, opposition to vaccines, quack science, and a lack of leadership are not what we need. This seems like a formula for pandemic disaster.

chapter thirty

Trump Attacks Harvard

To many, especially the cultural elite, Harvard University is the ultimate symbol of academic excellence. Nine former US presidents, beginning with John Adams, have Harvard degrees. Ten current senators, including four Republicans, have Harvard degrees. It is the oldest college in the United States and the most challenging for young people seeking admission. It has 20,000 employees and 20,000 students, but only about 7,000 of the students are undergraduates. The acceptance rate for applicants is about 4%.

Why Trump decided to attack Harvard with such vengeance has been questioned. Some speculated about the possibility that he or a family member may have been turned down for admittance;[207,208] there is no good evidence for this. A few prominent Democratic political leaders, like Vice President Gore and President and Mrs. Obama, as well as their children, were Harvard students, as were many children of prominent Republican families.

Another line of thinking is that Trump might be particularly vengeful toward Harvard because of the prominent role played by Penny Pritzker, the chair of Harvard's Corporation Board.[209,210] An heiress to the Hyatt Hotels fortune, she was the national finance chair of Obama's first presidential campaign and the secretary of commerce during his second administration. She is also the sister of J.B. Pritzker, the governor of Illinois, who may be a Democratic candidate for president in the future. Trump was involved in a major business deal with the Pritzker family decades ago in New York City. The deal failed, and Trump threatened retaliation:

"I always said, the first time I got back on my feet, the Pritzkers would be the first people I'd go after."[209]

Beyond personal retribution, it is easy to see why Trump might think that attacking Harvard might play well with his base. He once stated, "I love the poorly educated," suggesting a political strategy of anti-intellectualism and control over experts and expertise.[211,212] This is, of course, a major tenet in the autocrat playbook.

The administration and faculty at Harvard have evolved to become disproportionately liberal and progressive over the last 50 years. Only 3% of Harvard faculty describe their politics as conservative.[213] The children of prominent Republicans still go to Harvard, but they often feel culturally or socially isolated once there. This is probably true for most of the best universities in the United States, whether they are in Cambridge, Massachusetts, or Austin, Texas.

Some said Trump was targeting Harvard because it seemed like the best way to intimidate other universities to follow his worldview. Ty Cobb, a White House lawyer during Trump's first term, said that "he hates Harvard, and he wants to punish them however he can."[210] Trump soon found quite a few ways to use his government to punish Harvard. He believed he could take away federal research grant money and block the right of Harvard professors to apply for such funds in the future.[214] He could also mobilize the Department of Homeland Security to block visas for international students and research fellows who wished to train at Harvard.[215] Trump believed he could use the Internal Revenue Service to force higher taxes on Harvard's substantial endowment income.[216] He would also try to recover patent income related to discoveries by faculty who may have received government grant support.[217] Trump would also try to convince national or regional university regulatory agencies to take away Harvard's accreditation.[218] For all these actions, he would use the rationale of antisemitism and/or the presumption that Harvard inappropriately used diversity for their selection of both students and faculty.[216]

The first indication of concern about a problem with federal research grant funding at Harvard came when the government threatened to drastically reduce overhead reimbursements (or "indirect costs").[219] Overhead reimbursements normally go to the university to complement direct research funds. The overhead is used to pay expenses related to the laboratory space where the research is done. These include electricity, heating, and cleaning, as well as the accounting of grant expenditures.

While this was going on, the National Institutes of Health (NIH) was already blocking the funding of research on topics that conservative government officials found distasteful. These included grants on topics like the health problems of minority populations, gender issues, and vaccines.[220,221] This policy was not specific to Harvard, but the impact was substantial for Harvard investigators, especially faculty at the T.H. Chan School of Public Health (HSPH), who had numerous research programs on these topics. As you enter the school, a message engraved in the wall in multiple languages reads, "The highest attainable standard of health is one of the fundamental rights of every human being." It came from the preamble of the constitution of the World Health Organization.

By May 2025, the Trump administration notified Harvard that all research grants and contracts would be terminated immediately and future applications would not be considered.[216] The first government message was that $8.7 billion in funding was being reviewed for termination. This figure included about $6 billion that went to Harvard-affiliated faculty who are based at the associated hospitals and research institutes rather than at the university campus. The hospital-based funds were subsequently left alone, but the government did cancel almost $3 billion in grant funds that went directly to full-time Harvard faculty.

About 47% of the budget of HSPH, where I was based, is from the government, especially the US NIH, as is about one-third of the budget of the Harvard Medical School. These funds support research on a range of health topics, from cancer and heart disease to the cost-effectiveness of different methods of health-care delivery. Infectious diseases, including global epidemics, feature prominently in the agenda for HSPH. Most NIH grants are given for 5-year periods. So termination in years 3, 4, or 5 means that the financial and intellectual investments of all prior years may be wasted.

A long-term NIH-sponsored study to monitor the health of nurses and other health-care professionals has been in place at HSPH since 1980.[222] About 250,000 women have been followed for decades. For research purposes, it is a unique population resource. The study evaluates genetic and lifestyle factors to determine the causes of cancer, heart disease, and other illnesses. As new diagnostic tests and disease monitoring tools are discovered, it allows researchers to look back at blood samples stored long before to see which might best predict a particular outcome. New tests may then become available for cancer prevention, treatment, or early diagnosis. The termination of research projects such as this means that much of the previous work on the program may also be lost if there are no funds to maintain the frozen samples and the database.

The bludgeoning of NIH research is not only devastating for the scientists and the universities, it is also a major loss for health care and for the economy. It has been estimated that each dollar of NIH research generates three dollars of economic activity. Ninety-nine percent of drugs currently approved for use have had NIH funding.[223] According to the Nature Index guide for high-quality research in the sciences, Harvard ranks first worldwide among academic institutions. All others in the top 10 are in China.[224] Even before Trump's attacks on Harvard and the NIH, the number of drug trials done in China had increased sixfold in the last 5 years. Trump's attacks make it even more likely that China will replace the United States as the future world leader in research.

Soon after announcing his decision to block research funding at Harvard, Trump also declared that foreign students would no longer be able to come to the university.[216] To implement this, the Department of Homeland Security terminated Harvard's certification for the Student and Exchange Visitor Program. This blocked the ability of foreign applicants, whether students, research fellows, or visiting faculty, from getting visas to go to Harvard. Those already at Harvard would be forced to leave the country or go to a different university.

This action also had profound implications. Harvard is an international institution. About 27% of the students who attend Harvard are from other countries. This includes 15% of undergraduates,

37% of students at HSPH, and more than half at the Kennedy School of Government. About half of the postdoctoral research fellows at Harvard are from other countries. The Harvard International Office lists students and scholars coming from about 150 countries during the current year.

Having a large number of foreign students at a US university is not unique to Harvard. Quite a few US universities have 15% or more of their students coming from other countries. There are more than a million foreign students in US colleges, more than half coming from India or China. Some of the foreign students want to stay in the United States after their training period. This is good for our country, at least in relation to economic development. It has been estimated that 43% of our PhD-level workers in STEM (science, technology, engineering, mathematics)-related areas were foreign born,[225] as were half of the CEOs of the 10 largest US companies.

The main rationale given by the Trump administration for its attacks on Harvard was antisemitism and failing to keep Jewish students safe.[216] This was probably overblown, but it became an issue because of protests about the Israel–Gaza war. Harvard was also accused of discriminating against white people, Asian Americans, heterosexuals, and men,[226] and of working with China.

Harvard denied the accusations of discrimination, sued the government, and won in court, at least in the first round.[216] Harvard president Alan Garber conceded that antisemitism was an issue but insisted that Harvard was focused on the problem. Garber strongly resisted government demands to change policies on admissions, hiring, and governance, which were considered central to academic freedom.

For several decades while I was a faculty department chair at Harvard, we followed specific guidelines against discrimination. The guidelines required that women and racial minorities of equal merit be considered for new positions and promotions. I recall feeling a sense of accomplishment when we successfully recruited highly qualified women and members of racial minority groups. At least half the faculty members in our department were women, and the women were as successful as the men.

The current Harvard president, Alan Garber, and the chairperson of the Corporation Board, Penny Pritzker, are both Jews. About half of our department faculty members were Jews, though I don't ever recall anyone suggesting we must include Jews in our recruitment or hiring procedures. It just happened that way. While I was a department chair for about 25 years, I served under four deans and three university presidents. Six of the seven were Jews. During this time, no concerns were expressed to me about antisemitism from students, faculty, staff, or the administration. Having retired before the attack on Israel on October 7, 2023, I was less exposed to the student protests that came later. The Harvard medical campus, where I and most of the research are based, is in Boston, miles away from the undergraduate campus in Cambridge, where most of the protests took place. Regardless of the severity of the problem of antisemitism, the elimination of medical research does not seem to be a logical solution.

Harvard sued the Trump administration in federal court in April 2025 for freezing the research grants. In September, US District Judge Allison Burroughs ruled in Harvard's favor, stating that the Trump administration's freeze of federal research funds was unconstitutional, amounted to retaliation, and violated federal law. The administration may appeal. In May, the government revoked Harvard's ability to admit international students. The next day, Judge Burroughs stated that the government is barred from taking away Harvard's certification to enroll international students while a court challenge unfolds.[227]

Many legal experts believe Harvard has a strong case and should win in the end. But considerable damage has already been done. Medical experiments and clinical trials have been interrupted, and valuable results will be lost. Some of the best senior scientists will leave to work in places where their research will not be threatened. Young scientists will have their careers derailed. Many international students and research fellows will avoid Harvard and the United States. In October 2025, some of Harvard's NIH research grant funds were restored to the university, but there is concern that they could be blocked again pending the government's appeal.

Newly emerging infectious diseases that enter the human population in the future, as did the coronavirus in 2019 and HIV in the early 1980s, will probably cause more deaths and greater damage to the economy. Our knowledge about how to detect new viruses and new epidemics is much better. Our expertise for making vaccines and drugs is vastly improved. Our capacity to communicate public health knowledge is powerful. However, these advantages are more than offset by the current state of our damaged systems needed for human cooperation and collaboration. The US CDC, previously the leading source of knowledge about public health policy, has been decimated. The US NIH, the FDA, and our leading public health research centers have been similarly attacked and designated for major reductions in funding. Our networks for communication of public health information have been seriously contaminated with conspiracy theories and misinformation. The United States has withdrawn from the WHO and closed down sites for cooperation and aid in developing countries where such new infectious diseases usually begin. Our lag time for a successful response to HIV/AIDS was 10–15 years. For COVID, it was 2–3 years. For those epidemics, the United States was the driving force for saving lives in the American population and the world. For the next one, we may be dependent on China to play that role.

My own career began soon after our government, especially through the NIH and our universities, was undergoing a massive expansion in medical research. Long-term investments in basic research and training were expanding, along with a mentality for international cooperation. My retirement, about 50 years later, occurred just before the destruction of this system. I am enormously thankful for the opportunity I had to play a small role in this era of success, but sad that my most recent students will not have similar opportunities. However, I have even greater sadness for the national and global population, who will have to wait longer for each successful result, whether it is for the next epidemic or a cure for cancer.

Glossary

AAC AIDS Action Committee. A nonprofit organization established in Boston in 1983 to provide services, including health care, to AIDS patients.

ACTG 076 AIDS Clinical Trials Group protocol #076. The ACTG is a network of research organizations established by the US National Institutes of Health to conduct clinical trials on drugs for HIV/AIDS. The 076 study trial was done to determine if a particular drug, AZT, could lower the risk for HIV-infected mothers to infect their infants before or during birth.

ACT UP AIDS Coalition to Unleash Power. An activist group formed in 1987 to end the AIDS epidemic.

Adjuvant A substance that enhances the body's immune response to an antigen, such as a vaccine.

AFRIMS Armed Forces Research Institute of Medical Sciences. A collaborative organization between military researchers of the United States and Thailand to study diseases of joint interest.

AIDS Acquired immunodeficiency syndrome.

Amplifier host A species of bird or mammal that enhances the spread of a new epidemic agent of a type that might infect people, thereby increasing the risk of human infections.

Amyl nitrate poppers, butyl nitrate poppers Chemical drugs used in inhalers to produce euphoria, often used during sex.

Antibodies Protein substances produced by the body in response to foreign invaders such as viruses. Vaccines are usually designed to mimic a virus to induce protective antibodies.

Antigenic drift A situation seen with highly variable viruses where the virus surface rapidly changes, causing vaccine-induced antibodies to lose effectiveness rapidly.

Anti-vaxxers People who are opposed to the use of vaccines.

Aplastic anemia A blood disease characterized by an inability of the bone marrow to make enough blood cells.

ARV Antiretroviral. A medication used to treat or prevent a disease caused by a retrovirus, such as HIV.

ATL Adult T cell leukemia. A highly lethal form of leukemia caused by the human T cell leukemia virus.

AZT Azidothymidine, also called ZDV for zidovudine. The first drug that showed an effect against HIV. A reverse transcriptase inhibitor.

BCPP Botswana Combination Prevention Project, also known by the Setswana name "Ya Tsie." A research project designed by the Botswana Harvard Partnership (BHP) to evaluate the use of anti-HIV drugs and other prevention measures to reduce spread of HIV.

BHP Botswana Harvard Partnership, now known as the Botswana Harvard Health Partnership, formerly known as the Botswana Harvard AIDS Institute Partnership. Established in 1996 as a collaborative research and training partnership between the Botswana Ministry of Health and the Harvard AIDS Institute.

Biohazard level 3 A set of standards for a research laboratory to conduct experiments with dangerous infectious agents, especially certain viruses.

BL Burkitt lymphoma. A type of cancer associated with the Epstein-Barr virus. Frequently occurs in immunosuppressed people.

B lymphocytes Bone marrow-derived blood cells that make antibodies.

Butyl nitrate poppers See amyl nitrate poppers.

CAIDS Community-acquired immunodeficiency disease. A term used to describe the clinical disease AIDS in the early years of the epidemic, before the identification of HIV.

Candidiasis A yeast infection of mucosal surfaces that is common in patients with immunosuppression.

CCR5 A chemokine receptor on lymphocytes that serves as an attachment site for HIV when it infects cells.

CDC Centers for Disease Control and Prevention. A US governmental agency that monitors epidemics.

CD4 A receptor on lymphocytes that HIV attaches to when infecting cells.

Commensal A category of microbes, especially bacteria, that live in another living organism without causing harm. Bacteria in the intestines of people are an example.

Contact inhibition The mechanism by which normal cells stop proliferating when they touch other cells, whereas cancer cells are not inhibited.

Coronavirus A group of viruses characterized by surface spikes that resemble a crown. These viruses occur in various species and are associated with respiratory diseases in people.

COVID Coronavirus infectious disease. Often used to describe disease also called SARS.

Creutzfeldt-Jakob disease A neurodegenerative brain disorder.

CRF Circulating recombinant form. A new hybrid virus found in the blood of a person who was infected with two different "parental" viruses at the same time.

Cryptococcosis An infectious disease caused by yeast of Cryptococcus species. Often occurs in patients with advanced AIDS.

CSH Cold Spring Harbor Laboratory and Conference Center. A renowned biological research laboratory in New York.

Dane particle Hepatitis B virus as it may be found as complete particles in blood.

Dead-end host A person or animal who can get infected with a virus but does not transmit it to others.

Delta 32 A mutation in the CCR5 gene that makes cells difficult or impossible to infect with HIV.

Double blinded A clinical trial design to test a drug or vaccine in which neither the trial participants nor the research staff know whether any particular individual received the experimental drug/vaccine or a placebo.

Double helix The appearance of DNA as it exists in the chromosomes of cells.

DRC The Democratic Republic of Congo. Formerly called Zaire.

Ebola A rare but deadly virus that causes hemorrhagic fever, primarily in Africa.

EBV Epstein-Barr virus. The cause of a type of lymphoma that is common in AIDS patients.

EEE Eastern equine encephalitis. A serious mosquito-borne viral disease of horses and occasionally people in the eastern United States.

EFV Efavirenz. An antiretroviral drug used by AIDS patients.

Endemic A disease-causing virus or microbe that is regularly present in a particular population or country.

Endogenous virus Viral elements related to retroviruses that are present in normal human or animal DNA.

Endotoxin A toxin inside bacterial cells that is released when the bacteria die.

Epithelial cells Abundant cells that make up skin and the lining of body organs.

Equipoise To establish balance or equity – for example, between two different arms of a clinical trial.

Equivalence trial A clinical trial designed to determine whether a new drug or intervention is equal to another existing drug or intervention.

Factor VIII A protein needed for blood clotting that is lacking in hemophiliacs.

Factorial design A statistical design for a clinical trial that allows a comparison of multiple entities at the same time.

FDA Food and Drug Administration. A US government agency that approves drugs and vaccines based on safety and efficacy.

FeLV Feline leukemia virus.

FeSV Feline sarcoma virus.

Fitness advantage In genetics, the ability of a species, such as a virus, to survive better as a population in a particular environment.

Founder effect In epidemiology or population genetics, a particular organism, such as a virus, that dominates in a host population because it got there first and saturated a particular niche.

Gavi The Vaccine Alliance.

Gécamines A large mining company in the Democratic Republic of Congo.

Genome The complete set of genes that define a particular species.

Glomerulonephritis An infection or inflammation of the filtration cells in the kidney.

Glycoprotein A molecule made up of both protein and carbohydrate.

Gnotobiotic The study of animals in a germ-free environment.

gp61 A glycoprotein of 61,000 daltons that is found on the outer surface of HTLV virus particles.

gp120 A glycoprotein of 120,000 daltons that is found on the outer surface of HIV virus particles.

gp160 A glycoprotein of 160,000 daltons that is found on the outer surface of cells that are infected with HIV.

GRID Gay-related immunodeficiency disease. A term used to describe AIDS before the cause and scope of the disease were understood.

Group M The Major or Main group of HIV-1 viruses that had a common origin in chimpanzees.

HAART Highly active antiretroviral therapy. The use of several drugs against HIV used in combination that can reduce virus replication to negligible levels and restore health.

HAI Harvard AIDS Institute.

HBV Hepatitis B virus.

HeLa cells An immortalized cell culture line taken from cancer patient Henrietta Lacks in 1951, often used in laboratory research.

Hepatitis An infection or inflammation of the liver.

Herd immunity A situation where a large portion of the population is immune to an infectious agent by either vaccination or prior infection, greatly reducing the chance of infectious transmission.

Herpes saimiri A virus found naturally in healthy squirrel monkeys that may cause an aggressive leukemia when injected into some other species of monkeys.

Herpes zoster The virus that causes shingles and chickenpox in people.

HHV8 Human herpesvirus 8, also known as Kaposi sarcoma–associated herpesvirus (KSHV).

Hit and run theory A hypothesis by which some viruses may cause cancer and then disappear from the body by the time the cancer is detected.

HIV Human immunodeficiency virus. The virus that causes AIDS.

HIV/AIDS The AIDS disease caused by HIV.

HIV-1 The most common HIV virus. Responsible for the worldwide pandemic of AIDS.

HIV-1A, B, C, D, E Subtypes of HIV-1.

HIV-1 A/C, A/E, A/G Hybrid viruses generated from two different subtypes of HIV.

HIV-2 The second HIV discovered, found primarily in West Africa and less virulent than HIV-1.

Horseshoe bats The species of bats found in China that appear to be the natural host for the SARS-2 COVID virus.

Host cell receptor The protein on the surface of cells that allows attachment of a virus like HIV.

HPV Human papilloma virus. Some HPVs cause warts or epithelial cancers like cancer of the uterine cervix.

HSPH Harvard T.H. Chan School of Public Health.

HTLV, HTLV-I Human T cell leukemia virus. The cause of adult T cell leukemia.

HTLV-II A second human T cell virus related to HTLV-I.

HTLV-III The first name given to the virus that causes AIDS, before it was renamed HIV.

HTLV-III/LAV Another name for HIV-1 in the early years of discovery. Includes the lymphadenopathy-associated virus, which was shown to be the same as HTLV-III.

HTLV-IV The original name given to the virus that was later named HIV-2.

Hybrid virus A new virus shown to contain gene sequences from two or more parental viruses.

Hypertransmitter A virus-infected person who is highly infectious for others because of large amounts of virus in their mucosal fluids.

IAS International AIDS Society.

IDU Injection drug user.

Immunofluorescence A laboratory technique that uses an antibody attached to a fluorescent dye to allow visual detection of a particular molecule.

Immunogenic A molecule that can induce an immune response.

Immunogenicity The relative ability of an antigen, such as a vaccine, to induce an immune response.

Immunosurveillance A theory that newly arising cancer cells stimulate an immune response that eliminates a growing cancer.

Infectious agent A virus or other microbe that infects the body.

Infectious clone As used in virology, a set of viral genes that yields a homogeneous population of progeny virus in a laboratory cell culture.

Integrase An enzyme that retroviruses like HIV use to insert a copy of their genome into the cell DNA of the patient.

Killer T lymphocytes A type of blood cell that attacks and kills cells that present foreign substances, such as viruses.

KITSO An AIDS training program for health-care personnel developed in Botswana.

KS, Kaposi sarcoma A type of cancer of the skin or mucous membranes that occurs more frequently in patients with immunosuppression.

KSHV Kaposi sarcoma–associated herpesvirus.

Latency A period of delay or concealment that can occur after viral infection before the infection shows disease symptoms.

LAV Lymphadenopathy-associated virus. The first name given to HIV by French investigators when the virus was identified in patients with swollen lymph nodes.

LC Langerhans cells. Specialized cells of the immune system found in skin and mucosal tissues.

LGBTQ Lesbian, gay, bisexual, transgender, and queer.

Lymphoblast A precursor of lymphocytes found in bone marrow.

Lymphocytes Immune cells that circulate in the blood and are present in lymph nodes.

M Main or Major category of HIV-1 viruses.

Macaques A genus of old-world monkeys found in Asia.

Mad cow disease A neurological disease of cattle due to an abnormally folded protein called a prion.

Masked palm civet A small mammal in China that is sometimes used as bushmeat and is frequently infected with a COVID-type virus.

Meningitis An infection or inflammation of the tissues that cover the brain.

MERS Middle East respiratory syndrome. A viral disease similar to COVID that occurs in the Middle East and is most common in people who have close exposure to camels.

Messenger RNA A molecule of nucleic acid that translates a DNA gene code to make protein in cells.

MIT Massachusetts Institute of Technology.

MMR Measles, mumps, rubella.

Molnupiravir An antiviral drug used to treat COVID.

MS, multiple sclerosis A chronic disease of the central nervous system.

Mucosal cells Cells that line sites such as the mouth, pharynx, and reproductive organs and produce mucus as an antimicrobial defense.

Mutagenesis A laboratory procedure used by geneticists to select for mutations in genes.

Mycobacteria A genus of bacteria, some of which cause tuberculosis in people and animals.

Myeloproliferative disease A form of cancer due to malignant alteration of bone marrow progenitor cells.

NATO North Atlantic Treaty Organization.

NCI National Cancer Institute.

New Fore people Indigenous Peoples in Papua New Guinea that had cases of the disease kuru.

NIH National Institutes of Health. The government agency responsible for most medical research in the United States.

90–90–90 A UNAIDS goal to identify 90% of the people with HIV infection in a given country, to treat 90% of those with drugs, and to verify that 90% of those treated have low viral loads.

Ntlo ya Dikgosi A government advisory body of tribal chiefs in Botswana.

NVP, Nevirapine A drug used to inhibit HIV replication by interfering with the viral reverse transcription.

Omicron variant A new variant of COVID responsible for most cases of the disease. First identified in Botswana.

Oncogenes Genes, often captured by retroviruses, that can make cultured cells show cancerous properties.

PAHO Pan American Health Organization. A branch of the United Nations World Health Organization.

Pandemic A worldwide epidemic.

Papilloma virus A group of viruses in humans and other species that cause warts and carcinoma cancers.

Paroxysmal A sudden increase of disease symptoms.
Pathognomonic A sign or symptom that is particularly unique for a particular disease.
Paxlovid An antiviral drug that is used for COVID.
PCR Polymerase chain reaction. A very sensitive test that detects specific gene sequences.
PEP Post-exposure prophylaxis. The use of drugs to prevent infection as in the case of laboratory or medical personnel using anti-HIV drugs after an accidental needle stick.
PEPFAR US President's Emergency Plan for AIDS Relief.
Phenotype The observable traits and appearance associated with particular groups of living things.
Phlebotomist A medical worker trained to withdraw blood.
Phylogenetic The evolutionary relatedness between populations.
Placebo A harmless, inert drug or vaccine formulated for a clinical trial so those injected with an experimental drug cannot determine whether they were injected with the actual experimental material or an inert control substance.
Pneumocystis pneumonia A serious type of fungal pneumonia that occurs in people who have an impaired immune system.
Pre-AIDS A medical condition with swollen lymph nodes that HIV-infected patients often get before they develop the more lethal opportunistic infections and cancers associated with AIDS.
PrEP Pre-exposure prophylaxis. A procedure of taking anti-HIV drugs before potential exposure to HIV to prevent infection.
Prion A class of infectious protein molecules folded in abnormal ways that cause diseases like kuru and mad cow disease.
Prophylaxis Use of a prevention procedure to avoid infection or disease.
Protease inhibitor An antiviral drug that targets the protease that some viruses, like HIV, need for infection.
PWA Person with AIDS.
Raccoon dog A fox-like wild animal in Asia that was a candidate for transmitting COVID to people.
Radioimmunoprecipitation A laboratory technique using antibodies and radioactively labeled cells to identify specific proteins.
Radiolabel amino acid sequencing A technique that uses isotopes to identify proteins using knowledge of the gene sequence.
Reassortment A process by which one type of flu virus exchanges genes with a different flu virus when both infect the same cell, resulting in hybrid progeny viruses that can then seed a new epidemic.
Recombinant progeny virus A hybrid virus found in a person who got infected with two discernibly different parental viruses.

Replication cycle The time period between when a virus infects a cell and when it releases progeny viruses to infect other cells.

Retrovirus A class of viruses like HIV that have a necessary step for copying the viral RNA genome into DNA and inserting that DNA into the infected cell.

Reverse transcription The process by which retroviruses copy their viral RNA into DNA.

RNA Ribonucleic acid. The molecule that viruses like HIV and COVID use as their viral genome.

R0 A reproductive number that measures how transmissible an infectious agent may be in a particular population.

Sarc A cancer-related gene and protein initially identified in some chicken retroviruses.

Sarcoma A type of tumor that occurs in bone and muscle.

SARS; SARS 1, 2 Severe acute respiratory syndrome. Same as COVID.

SARS-CoV-1 The SARS COVID virus and epidemic first observed in 2002–2004.

SARS-CoV-2 The SARS COVID virus and epidemic first observed in 2019.

Scrapie An infectious disease of sheep caused by abnormally folded proteins; related to mad cow disease and kuru.

Setswana The language spoken by the Tswana people of Botswana and South Africa.

Shoe leather epidemiology Looking for the cause of a disease by studying disease cases, their environment, and their contacts.

Site-specific mutagenesis A laboratory technique to make mutations in a particular spot in DNA to observe the effects on gene function.

SIV Simian immunodeficiency virus.

Spillover In the context of infectious diseases, the transfer of a virus from an animal species to humans.

STEM Science, technology, engineering, mathematics.

Sterilizing immunity A type of immunity that is so efficient it does not allow the infectious agent to infect the host and allow transmission.

STLV Simian T cell lymphotropic virus. A retrovirus of monkeys found in association with T cell leukemia.

STLV-III Simian T cell lymphotropic virus. A virus of monkeys associated with immunosuppression and related to HTLV-III of people. Later renamed SIV-1.

Subtype A subset of HIVs based on genetic relatedness. Different subtypes may be responsible for different regional epidemics within the world pandemic.

TasP Treatment as prevention. The approach of screening populations of people for HIV and treating all HIV-positive people to reduce the number of people who can transmit the virus.

T cells Lymphocytes in the immune system that program immune responses.

T4 Subgroup of T cells. Same as T helper cells.

T4 lymphocytes Cells that trigger the immune system to mount a positive response.

T helper cells Lymphocytes that are required for adaptive immune responses.

3x5 Program A plan by UNAIDS introduced in 2003 with a goal of treating 3 million people with HIV/AIDS by 2005.

Togavirus A family of RNA viruses that are often transmitted by mosquitoes.

Transcription The process by which living cells copy their genes or genomes.

Transduction A laboratory procedure for introducing pure DNA into a cell to understand gene function.

Transformation A laboratory procedure to make cells acquire the characteristics of cancer cells.

TSP Tropical spastic paraparesis. A neurological disease associated with HTLV infection.

T suppressor cells A type of immune regulator cell that keeps the immune system from overreacting.

Typhoid Mary A person who is believed to be highly efficient in transmitting an infectious disease.

UCD University of California at Davis.

UCLA University of California at Los Angeles.

UCSF University of California at San Francisco.

Ultracentrifuge A laboratory instrument that creates extremely high gravitation force. Used to concentrate small particles like viruses.

UNAIDS Joint United Nations Programme on HIV/AIDS.

USAID United States Agency for International Development.

VEE Venezuelan equine encephalitis virus.

Viral genetic linkage mapping The use of viral genome sequences to determine the relative location of genetic markers.

Viremia The presence of virus in the blood of an infected person or animal.

Viremic A person with viremia.

VL, viral load The amount of virus in the blood of an infected person.

Wasting A condition of emaciation seen in some patients with advanced chronic diseases such as AIDS or cancer.

Wet market A market that sells fresh meat, often referring to markets in Asia and Africa that sell animals caught in the wild.

WHO World Health Organization. A branch of the United Nations.

WSU Washington State University.

Xenotropic A virus that proliferates best in species other than the one in which it is naturally found in the DNA.

Ya Tsie The village-based treatment as prevention trial for HIV in Botswana (see BCPP). A Setswana phrase meaning "together we can."

ZDV Zidovudine, the first drug widely used for treatment of HIV/AIDS. Same as AZT.

Zoonotic, zoonosis An infectious disease of people that was transmitted from lower animals.

References

1. Dickerman RW, Scherer WF, Moorhouse AS, Toaz E, Essex ME, Steele RE. Ecologic studies of Venezuelan encephalitis virus in southeastern Mexico. VI. Infection of wild birds. Am J Trop Med Hyg. 1972;21:66–78.
2. Scherer WF, Dickerman RW, Jordan EK, Saidi S, Zarate ML, Ventura AK. Ecologic studies of Venezuelan encephalitis virus in southeastern Mexico. II. Prevalance, and geographic and temporal distribution of virus measured by sentinel hamsters and mice. Am J Trop Med Hyg. 1971;20:740–53.
3. Scherer WF, Dickerman RW, Wong-Chia C, Ventura A, Moorhouse A, Geiger R, Diza Najera A. Venezuelan equine encephalitis virus in Veracruz, Mexico, and the use of hamsters as sentinels. Science. 1964;145:274–5.
4. Hu Z, Shi Z. Investigation of animal reservoir(s) of SARS-CoV. In: Lu Y, Essex M, Roberts B, editors. Emerging infections in Asia. New York: Springer; 2008. p. 57–73.
5. Essex M. The antibody response in conventional and germfree animals to heated and unheated whole milk [MS thesis]. East Lansing: Michigan State University; 1967.
6. Gross L. Oncogenic viruses. 2nd ed. Oxford: Pergamon Press; 1970.
7. Temin HM, Mizutani S. RNA-dependent DNA polymerase in virions of Rous sarcoma virus. Nature. 1970;226:1211–3.
8. Baltimore D. RNA-dependent DNA polymerase in virions of RNA tumour viruses. Nature. 1970;226:1209–11.
9. Snyder SP, Theilen GH. Transmissible feline fibrosarcoma. Nature. 1969;221:1074–5.

10. Kawakami TG, Huff SD, Buckley PM, Dungworth DL, Synder SP, Gilden RV. C-type virus associated with gibbon lymphosarcoma. Nat New Biol. 1972;235:170–1.
11. Theilen GH, Gould D, Fowler M, Dungworth DL. C-type virus in tumor tissue of a woolly monkey (Lagothrix spp.) with fibrosarcoma. J Natl Cancer Inst. 1971;47:881–9.
12. Jarrett WF, Crawford EM, Martin WB, Davie F. A virus-like particle associated with leukemia (lymphosarcoma). Nature. 1964;202:567–9.
13. Kawakami TG, Theilen GH, Dungworth DL, Munn RJ, Beall SG. "C"-type viral particles in plasma of cats with feline leukemia. Science. 1967;158:1049–50.
14. Watson JD. The double helix: a personal acount of the discovery of the structure of DNA. New York: Scribner; 1998.
15. Maxam AM, Gilbert W. A new method for sequencing DNA. Proc Natl Acad Sci U S A. 1977;74:560–4. PMCID: PMC392330.
16. Mullis K, Faloona F, Scharf S, Saiki R, Horn G, Erlich H. Specific enzymatic amplification of DNA in vitro: the polymerase chain reaction. Cold Spring Harb Symp Quant Biol. 1986;51 Pt 1:263–73.
17. Epstein MA, Achong BG, Barr YM. Virus particles in cultured lymphoblasts from Burkitt's lymphoma. Lancet. 1964;1:702–3.
18. Chang Y, Cesarman E, Pessin MS, Lee F, Culpepper J, Knowles DM, Moore PS. Identification of herpesvirus-like DNA sequences in AIDS-associated Kaposi's sarcoma. Science. 1994;266:1865–9.
19. Melendez LV, Daniel MD, Hunt RD, Garcia FG. An apparently new herpesvirus from primary kidney cultures of the squirrel monkey (Saimiri sciureus). Lab Anim Care. 1968;18:374–81.
20. Klein G. Confronting the holocaust: an eyewitness account. In: Braham RL, vanden Heuvel WJ, editors. The Auschwitz reports and the holocaust in Hungary. Boulder: Social Science Monographs; Rosenthal Institute for Holocaust Studies Graduate Center, City University of New York; 2011.
21. Essex M, Klein G, Snyder SP, Harrold JB. Correlation between humoral antibody and regression of tumours induced by feline sarcoma virus. Nature. 1971;233:195–6.
22. Essex M, Klein G, Snyder SP, Harrold JB. Antibody to feline oncornavirus-associated cell membrane antigen in neonatal cats. Int J Cancer. 1971;8:384–90.
23. Essex M, Sliski A, Cotter SM, Jakowski RR, Hardy WD Jr. Immunosurveillance of naturally occurring feline leukemia. Science. 1975;190:790–2.

24. Rosenberg M. Howard Hiatt: how this extraordinary mentor transformed health with science and compassion. Cambridge (MA): MIT Press; 2018.
25. Huebner RJ, Gilden RV. Inherited viral genomes (virogenes and oncogenes) in the etiology of cancer. In: Emmelot P, Bentvelzen P, editors. RNA viruses and host genome in oncogenesis. Amsterdam: North-Holland Publishing Co; 1972.
26. Cotter SM, Essex M, Hardy WD Jr. Serological studies of normal and leukemic cats in a multiple-case leukemia cluster. Cancer Res. 1974;34:1061–9.
27. Essex M, Jakowski RM, Hardy WD Jr, Cotter SM, Hess P, Sliski A. Feline oncornavirus-associated cell membrane antigen. III. Antibody titers in cats from leukemia cluster households. J Natl Cancer Inst. 1975;54:637–41.
28. Hardy WD Jr, McClelland AJ, Zuckerman EE, Hess PW, Essex M, Cotter SM, MacEwen EG, Hayes AA. Prevention of the contagious spread of feline leukaemia virus and the development of leukaemia in pet cats. Nature. 1976;263:326–8.
29. Essex M. Horizontally and vertically transmitted oncornaviruses of cats. Adv Cancer Res. 1975;21:175–248.
30. Jarrett W, Jarrett O, Mackey L, Laird H, Hardy W Jr, Essex M. Horizontal transmission of leukemia virus and leukemia in the cat. J Natl Cancer Inst. 1973;51:833–41.
31. Perryman LE, Hoover EA, Yohn DS. Immunologic reactivity of the cat: immunosuppression in experimental feline leukemia. J Natl Cancer Inst. 1972;49:1357–65.
32. Trainin Z, Wernicke D, Ungar-Waron H, Essex M. Suppression of the humoral antibody response in natural retrovirus infections. Science. 1983;220:858–9.
33. Skloot R. The immortal life of Henrietta Lacks. New York: Crown Publishers; 2010.
34. Stephenson JR, Essex M, Hino S, Hardy WD Jr, Aaronson SA. Feline oncornavirus-associated cell-membrane antigen (FOCMA): distinction between FOCMA and the major virion glycoprotein. Proc Natl Acad Sci U S A. 1977;74:1219–23. PMCID: PMC430654.
35. Sliski AH, Essex M, Meyer C, Todaro G. Feline oncornavirus-associated cell membrane antigen: expression in transformed nonproducer mink cells. Science. 1977;196:1336–9.
36. Gallo R. Virus hunting: AIDS, cancer, and the human retrovirus: a story of scientific discovery. New York: Basic Books; 1991.
37. Poiesz BJ, Ruscetti FW, Gazdar AF, Bunn PA, Minna JD, Gallo RC. Detection and isolation of type C retrovirus particles from fresh and

cultured lymphocytes of a patient with cutaneous T-cell lymphoma. Proc Natl Acad Sci U S A. 1980;77:7415–9. PMCID: PMC350514.
38. Uchiyama T, Yodoi J, Sagawa K, Takatsuki K, Uchino H. Adult T-cell leukemia: clinical and hematologic features of 16 cases. Blood. 1977;50:481–92.
39. Gessain A, Barin F, Vernant JC, Gout O, Maurs L, Calender A, de The G. Antibodies to human T-lymphotropic virus type-I in patients with tropical spastic paraparesis. Lancet. 1985;2:407–10.
40. Lee TH, Coligan JE, McLane MF, Sodroski JG, Popovic M, Wong-Staal F, Gallo RC, Haseltine W, Essex M. Serological cross-reactivity between envelope gene products of type I and type II human T-cell leukemia virus. Proc Natl Acad Sci U S A. 1984;81:7579–83. PMCID: PMC392190.
41. Lee TH, Coligan JE, Sodroski JG, Haseltine WA, Salahuddin SZ, Wong-Staal F, Gallo RC, Essex M. Antigens encoded by the 3′-terminal region of human T-cell leukemia virus: evidence for a functional gene. Science. 1984;226:57–61.
42. Homma T, Kanki PJ, King NW Jr, Hunt RD, O'Connell MJ, Letvin NL, Daniel MD, Desrosiers RC, Yang CS, Essex M. Lymphoma in macaques: association with virus of human T lymphotrophic family. Science. 1984;225:716–8.
43. Watson JD. The double helix. New York: Atheneum Press; 1968.
44. Dürst M, Gissmann L, Ikenberg H, zur Hausen H. A papillomavirus DNA from a cervical carcinoma and its prevalence in cancer biopsy samples from different geographic regions. Proc Natl Acad Sci U S A. 1983;80:3812–5. PMCID: PMC394142.
45. Essex M, Todaro G, zur Hausen H. Viruses in naturally occurring cancers. Books A and B. Cold Spring Harbor (NY): Cold Spring Harbor Laboratory Press; 1980.
46. Gallo RC, Essex M, Gross L. Human T cell leukemia/lymphoma virus. Cold Spring Harbor (NY): Cold Spring Harbor Laboratory Press; 1984.
47. Macleod IJ, O'Donnell B, Moyo S, Lockman S, Shapiro RL, Kayembe M, van Widenfelt E, Makhema J, Essex M, Wester C. Prevalence of human papillomavirus genotypes and associated cervical squamous intraepithelial lesions in HIV-infected women in Botswana. J Med Virol. 2011;83:1689–95. PMCID: PMC3156037.
48. Sahasrabuddhe VV, Mwanahamuntu MH, Vermund SH, Huh WK, Lyon MD, Stringer JSA, Parham GP. Prevalence and distribution of HPV genotypes among HIV-infected women in Zambia. Br J Cancer. 2007;96:1480–3. PMCID: PMC2360194.
49. Patel PR, Berenson AB. Sources of HPV vaccine hesitancy in parents. Hum Vaccin Immunother. 2013;9:2649–53. PMCID: PMC4162068.

50. Garolla A, Graziani A, Grande G, Ortolani C, Ferlin A. HPV-related diseases in male patients: an underestimated conundrum. J Endocrinol Invest. 2024;47:261–74. PMCID: PMC10859347.
51. Beral V, Jaffe H, Weiss R. Overview: cancer, HIV and AIDS. Cancer Surv. 1991;10:1–3.
52. Romet-Lemonne JL, Elfassi E, Haseltine W, Essex M. Infection of bone marrow cells by hepatitis B virus. Lancet. 1983;2:732.
53. Sureau C, Romet-Lemonne JL, Mullins JI, Essex M. Production of hepatitis B virus by a differentiated human hepatoma cell line after transfection with cloned circular HBV DNA. Cell. 1986;47:37–47.
54. Roingeard P, Diouf A, Sankale JL, Boye C, Mboup S, Diadhiou F, Essex M. Perinatal transmission of hepatitis B virus in Senegal, west Africa. Viral Immunol. 1993;6:65–73.
55. Gottlieb MS, Schroff R, Schanker HM, Weisman JD, Fan PT, Wolf RA, Saxon A. *Pneumocystis carinii* pneumonia and mucosal candidiasis in previously healthy homosexual men: evidence of a new acquired cellular immunodeficiency. N Engl J Med. 1981;305:1425–31.
56. Shilts R. And the band played on: politics, people, and the AIDS epidemic. New York: St Martin's Press; 1987.
57. Rogers MF, Morens DM, Stewart JA, Kaminski RM, Spira TJ, Feorino PM, Larsen SA, Francis DP, Wilson M, Kaufman L. National case-control study of Kaposi's sarcoma and *Pneumocystis carinii* pneumonia in homosexual men: Part 2. Laboratory results. Ann Intern Med. 1983;99:151–8.
58. Essex M, McLane MF, Lee TH, Falk L, Howe CW, Mullins JI, Cabradilla C, Francis DP. Antibodies to cell membrane antigens associated with human T-cell leukemia virus in patients with AIDS. Science. 1983;220:859–62.
59. Gelmann EP, Popovic M, Blayney D, Masur H, Sidhu G, Stahl RE, Gallo RC. Proviral DNA of a retrovirus, human T-cell leukemia virus, in two patients with AIDS. Science. 1983;220:862–5.
60. Gallo RC, Sarin PS, Gelmann EP, Robert-Guroff M, Richardson E, Kalyanaraman VS, Mann D, Sidhu GD, Stahl RE, Zolla-Pazner S, Leibowitch J, Popovic M. Isolation of human T-cell leukemia virus in acquired immune deficiency syndrome (AIDS). Science. 1983;220:865–7.
61. Barré-Sinoussi F, Chermann JC, Rey F, Nugeyre MT, Chamaret S, Gruest J, Dauguet C, Axler-Blin C, Vézinet-Brun F, Rouzioux C, Rozenbaum W, Montagnier L. Isolation of a T-lymphotropic retrovirus from a patient at risk for acquired immune deficiency syndrome (AIDS). Science. 1983;220:868–71.

62. Essex ME, McLane MF, Tachibana N, Francis DP, Lee TH. Seroepidemiology of human T-cell leukemia virus in relation to immunosuppression and the acquired immunodeficiency syndrome. In: Gallo RC, Essex ME, Gross L, editors. Human T-cell leukemia/lymphoma viruses. Cold Spring Harbor (NY): Cold Spring Harbor Laboratory; 1984. p. 355–62.
63. Essex M, McLane MF, Lee TH, Tachibana N, Mullins JI, Kreiss J, Kasper CK, Poon MC, Landay A, Stein SF, et al. Antibodies to human T-cell leukemia virus membrane antigens (HTLV-MA) in hemophiliacs. Science. 1983;221:1061–4.
64. Jaffe HW, Francis DP, McLane MF, Cabradilla C, Curran JW, Kilbourne BW, Lawrence DN, Haverkos HW, Spira TJ, Dodd RY, et al. Transfusion-associated AIDS: serologic evidence of human T-cell leukemia virus infection of donors. Science. 1984;223:1309–12.
65. Lee TH, Coligan JE, Homma T, McLane MF, Tachibana N, Essex M. Human T-cell leukemia virus-associated membrane antigens: identity of the major antigens recognized after virus infection. Proc Natl Acad Sci U S A. 1984;81:3856–60. PMCID: PMC345320.
66. Popovic M, Sarngadharan MG, Read E, Gallo RC. Detection, isolation, and continuous production of cytopathic retroviruses (HTLV-III) from patients with AIDS and pre-AIDS. Science. 1984;224:497–500.
67. Sarngadharan MG, Popovic M, Bruch L, Schüpbach J, Gallo RC. Antibodies reactive with human T-lymphotropic retroviruses (HTLV-III) in the serum of patients with AIDS. Science. 1984;224:506–8.
68. Schüpbach J, Popovic M, Gilden RV, Gonda MA, Sarngadharan MG, Gallo RC. Serological analysis of a subgroup of human T-lymphotropic retroviruses (HTLV-III) associated with AIDS. Science. 1984;224:503–5.
69. Gallo RC, Salahuddin SZ, Popovic M, Shearer GM, Kaplan M, Haynes BF, Palker TJ, Redfield R, Oleske J, Safai B, et al. Frequent detection and isolation of cytopathic retroviruses (HTLV-III) from patients with AIDS and at risk for AIDS. Science. 1984;224:500–3.
70. Kitchen LW, Barin F, Sullivan JL, McLane MF, Brettler DB, Levine PH, Essex M. Aetiology of AIDS – antibodies to human T-cell leukaemia virus (type III) in haemophiliacs. Nature. 1984;312:367–9.
71. Kreiss JK, Kitchen LW, Prince HE, Kasper CK, Essex M. Antibody to human T-lymphotropic virus type III in wives of hemophiliacs: evidence for heterosexual transmission. Ann Intern Med. 1985;102:623–6.
72. Allan JS, Coligan JE, Barin F, McLane MF, Sodroski JG, Rosen CA, Haseltine WA, Lee TH, Essex M. Major glycoprotein antigens that induce antibodies in AIDS patients are encoded by HTLV-III. Science. 1985;228:1091–4.

73. Barin F, McLane MF, Allan JS, Lee TH, Groopman JE, Essex M. Virus envelope protein of HTLV-III represents major target antigen for antibodies in AIDS patients. Science. 1985;228:1094–6.
74. Kanki PJ, Barin F, M'Boup S, Allan JS, Romet-Lemonne JL, Marlink R, McLane MF, Lee TH, Arbeille B, Denis F, et al. New human T-lymphotropic retrovirus related to simian T-lymphotropic virus type III (STLV-IIIAGM). Science. 1986;232:238–43.
75. Kanki PJ, Alroy J, Essex M. Isolation of T-lymphotropic retrovirus related to HTLV-III/LAV from wild-caught African green monkeys. Science. 1985;230:951–4.
76. Essex M. Human immunodeficiency viruses in the developing world. Adv Virus Res. 1999;53:71–88.
77. Shapiro RL, Thior I, Gilbert PB, Lockman S, Wester C, Smeaton LM, Stevens L, Heymann SJ, Ndung'u T, Gaseitsiwe S, et al. Maternal single-dose nevirapine versus placebo as part of an antiretroviral strategy to prevent mother-to-child HIV transmission in Botswana. AIDS. 2006;20:1281–8.
78. Thior I, Lockman S, Smeaton LM, Shapiro RL, Wester C, Heymann SJ, Gilbert PB, Stevens L, Peter T, Kim S, et al. Breastfeeding plus infant zidovudine prophylaxis for 6 months vs formula feeding plus infant zidovudine for 1 month to reduce mother-to-child HIV transmission in Botswana: a randomized trial: the Mashi Study. JAMA. 2006;296:794–805.
79. Essex M, Mboup S, Kanki PJ, Marlink RG, Tlou SD, editors. AIDS in Africa. 2nd ed. New York: Kluwer Academic/Plenum Publishers; 2002.
80. Kanki PJ, McLane MF, King NW Jr, Letvin NL, Hunt RD, Sehgal P, Daniel MD, Desrosiers RC, Essex M. Serologic identification and characterization of a macaque T-lymphotropic retrovirus closely related to HTLV-III. Science. 1985;228:1199–201.
81. Kanki PJ, Kurth R, Becker W, Dreesman G, McLane MF, Essex M. Antibodies to simian T-lymphotropic retrovirus type III in African green monkeys and recognition of STLV-III viral proteins by AIDS and related sera. Lancet. 1985;1:1330–2.
82. Quammen D. Spillover: animal infections and the next human pandemic. New York: W.W. Norton; 2012.
83. Gostin LO, Gronvall GK. The origins of Covid-19: why it matters (and why it doesn't). N Engl J Med. 2023;388:2305–8.
84. Kanki PJ, Travers KU, Mboup S, Hsieh CC, Marlink RG, Gueye-NDiaye A, Siby T, Thior I, Hernandez-Avila M, Sankalé JL, et al. Slower heterosexual spread of HIV-2 than HIV-1. Lancet. 1994;343:943–6.

85. Marlink R, Kanki P, Thior I, Travers K, Eisen G, Siby T, Traore I, Hsieh CC, Dia MC, Gueye EH, et al. Reduced rate of disease development after HIV-2 infection as compared to HIV-1. Science. 1994;265:1587–90.
86. Travers K, Mboup S, Marlink R, Guèye-Nidaye A, Siby T, Thior I, Traore I, Dieng-Sarr A, Sankalé JL, Mullins C, et al. Natural protection against HIV-1 infection provided by HIV-2. Science. 1995;268:1612–5.
87. Ornstein C, Costello D. A mother's denial, a daughter's death. Los Angeles Times [Internet]. 24 Sep 2005 [cited 2025 Oct 21]. Available from: https://www.latimes.com/archives/la-xpm-2005-sep-24-me-eliza24-story.html
88. Duesberg PH. Retroviruses as carcinogens and pathogens: expectations and reality. Cancer Res. 1987;47:1199–220.
89. Duesberg PH. Infectious AIDS: have we been misled? Berkeley (CA): North Atlantic Books; 1995.
90. Manjoo F. It's not possible to "win" an argument with Robert F. Kennedy Jr. New York Times [Internet]. 23 June 2023 [cited 2025 Oct 21]. Available from: https://www.nytimes.com/2023/06/23/opinion/rfk-jr-joe-rogan.html
91. Adams J. AIDS: the HIV myth. New York: St. Martin's Press; 1989.
92. Kalichman SC. Denying AIDS: conspiracy theories, pseudoscience, and human tragedy. Nattrass N, editor. New York: Copernicus/Springer; 2009.
93. Altman LK. U.N. official assails South Africa on its response to AIDS. New York Times [Internet]. 19 Aug 2006 [cited 2025 Oct 21]. Available from: https://www.nytimes.com/2006/08/19/world/africa/19aids.html
94. Chigwedere P, Essex M. AIDS denialism and public health practice. AIDS Behav. 2010;14:237–47.
95. Chigwedere P, Seage GR III, Gruskin S, Lee TH, Essex M. Estimating the lost benefits of antiretroviral drug use in South Africa. J Acquir Immune Defic Syndr. 2008;49:410–5.
96. Duesberg PH, Mandrioli D, McCormack A, Nicholson JM, Rasnick D, Fiala C, Koehnlein C, Bauer HH, Ruggiero M. AIDS since 1984: no evidence for a new, viral epidemic – not even in Africa. Ital J Anat Embryol. 2011;116:73–92.
97. Deer B. How the case against the MMR vaccine was fixed. BMJ. 2011;342:c5347.
98. Cohen J. Shots in the dark: the wayward search for an AIDS vaccine. New York: Norton; 2001.

99. Novitsky V, Gilbert P, Peter T, McLane MF, Gaolekwe S, Rybak N, Thior I, Ndung'u T, Marlink R, Lee TH, Essex M. Association between virus-specific T-cell responses and plasma viral load in human immunodeficiency virus type 1 subtype C infection. J Virol. 2003;77:882–90. PMCID: PMC140844.
100. Ndung'u T, Lu Y, Renjifo B, Touzjian N, Kushner N, Pena-Cruz V, Novitsky VA, Lee TH, Essex M. Infectious simian/human immunodeficiency virus with human immunodeficiency virus type 1 subtype C from an African isolate: rhesus macaque model. J Virol. 2001;75:11417–25. PMCID: PMC114728.
101. Essex M. The HIV-1 vaccine dilemma: lessons from the cat. J NIH Res. 1995;7:37–42.
102. Dow U, Essex M. Saturday is for funerals. Cambridge (MA): Harvard University Press; 2010.
103. Wallace J, Goldsmith-Pinkham P, Schwartz JL. Excess death rates for Republican and Democratic registered voters in Florida and Ohio during the COVID-19 pandemic. JAMA Intern Med. 2023;183:916–23. PMCID: PMC10366951.
104. Cherry JD, Krogstad P. SARS: the first pandemic of the 21st century. Pediatr Res. 2004;56:1–5. PMCID: PMC7086556.
105. Lu Y, Essex M, Roberts B. Emerging infections in Asia. New York: Springer Nature; 2008.
106. Yu D, Li H, Xu R, He J. Prevalence of IgG antibody to SARS-associated coronavirus in animal traders – Guangdong Province, China, 2003. MMWR Morb Mortal Wkly Rep. 2003;52:986–7.
107. Marra MA, Jones SJ, Astell CR, Holt RA, Brooks-Wilson A, Butterfield YS, Khattra J, Asano JK, Barber SA, Chan SY, et al. The genome sequence of the SARS-associated coronavirus. Science. 2003;300: 1399–404.
108. Zumla A, Hui DS, Perlman S. Middle East respiratory syndrome. Lancet. 2015;386:995–1007. PMCID: PMC4721578.
109. Pustake M, Tambolkar I, Giri P, Gandhi C. SARS, MERS and CoVID-19: an overview and comparison of clinical, laboratory and radiological features. J Family Med Prim Care. 2022;11:10–7. PMCID: PMC8930171.
110. Quammen D. The ongoing mystery of covid's origin. New York Times [Internet]. 18 Aug 2023 [cited 2023 Sep 26]. Available from: https://www.nytimes.com/2023/07/25/magazine/covid-start.html
111. Taylor A. Experts debunk fringe theory linking China's coronavirus to weapons research. Washington Post [Internet]. 29 Jan 2020 [cited 2023

Sep 26]. https://www.washingtonpost.com/world/2020/01/29/experts-debunk-fringe-theory-linking-chinas-coronavirus-weapons-research/
112. Editorial Board. In Wuhan, doctors knew the truth. They were told to keep quiet. Washington Post [Internet]. 22 Aug 2023 [cited 2023 Sep 26]. https://www.washingtonpost.com/opinions/2023/08/22/wuhan-doctors-pandemic-china-coverup/
113. Barin F, M'Boup S, Denis F, Kanki P, Allan JS, Lee TH, Essex M. Serological evidence for virus related to simian T-lymphotropic retrovirus III in residents of west Africa. Lancet. 1985;2:1387–9.
114. Nahmias AJ, Weiss J, Yao X, Lee F, Kodsi R, Schanfield M, Matthews T, Bolognesi D, Durack D, Motulsky A, Kanki P, Essex M. Evidence for human infection with an HTLV III/LAV-like virus in Central Africa, 1959. Lancet. 1986;1:1279–80.
115. Zhu T, Korber BT, Nahmias AJ, Hooper E, Sharp PM, Ho DD. An African HIV-1 sequence from 1959 and implications for the origin of the epidemic. Nature. 1998;391:594–7.
116. Pepin J. The origins of AIDS. Cambridge: Cambridge University Press; 2011.
117. Essex M. HIV/AIDS. In: Kirch W, editor. Encyclopedia of public health. New York: Springer; 2008.
118. Anderson KC, Gorgone BC, Marlink RG, Ferriani R, Essex ME, Benz PM, Groopman JE. Transfusion-acquired human immunodeficiency virus infection among immunocompromised persons. Ann Intern Med. 1986;105:519–27.
119. Renjifo B, Chaplin B, Mwakagile D, Shah P, Vannberg F, Msamanga G, Hunter D, Fawzi W, Essex M. Epidemic expansion of HIV type 1 subtype C and recombinant genotypes in Tanzania. AIDS Res Hum Retroviruses. 1998;14:635–8.
120. Yarchoan R, Mitsuya H, Broder S. AIDS therapies. Sci Am. 1988;259:110–9.
121. Bangsberg DR. A paradigm shift to prevent HIV drug resistance. PLoS Med. 2008;5:e111. PMCID: PMC2386833.
122. Brenner BG, Oliveira M, Doualla-Bell F, Moisi DD, Ntemgwa ML, Frankel FA, Essex M, Wainberg MA. HIV-1 subtype C viruses rapidly develop K65R resistance to tenofovir in cell culture. AIDS. 2006;20:F9–13.
123. Smith MW, Dean M, Carrington M, Huttley GA, O'Brien SJ. CCR5-delta 32 gene deletion in HIV-1 infected patients. Lancet. 1997;350:741.
124. Matsuda Z, Yu X, Yu QC, Lee TH, Essex M. A virion-specific inhibitory molecule with therapeutic potential for human immunodeficiency

virus type 1. Proc Natl Acad Sci U S A. 1993;90:3544–8. PMCID: PMC46337.

125. Essex M. Subtypes, strains, recombination, and reinfection: clinical and epidemiological relevance. In: Kanki PJ, Marlink RG, editors. A line drawn in the sand. Cambridge (MA): Harvard University Press; 2009. p. 245–58.
126. Soto-Ramirez LE, Renjifo B, McLane MF, Marlink R, O'Hara C, Sutthent R, Wasi C, Vithayasai P, Vithayasai V, Apichartpiyakul C, et al. HIV-1 Langerhans' cell tropism associated with heterosexual transmission of HIV. Science. 1996;271:1291–3.
127. Cohen J. Differences in HIV strains may underlie disease patterns. Science. 1995;270:30–1.
128. Rojanapithayakorn W, Hanenberg R. The 100% condom program in Thailand. AIDS. 1996;10:1–7.
129. Tripathy SP. History of HIV in India. In: Lu Y, Essex M, editors. AIDS in Asia. New York: Springer; 2004. p. 37–46.
130. Tripathy S, Renjifo B, Wang WK, McLane MF, Bollinger R, Rodrigues J, Osterman J, Tripathy S, Essex M. Envelope glycoprotein 120 sequences of primary HIV type 1 isolates from Pune and New Delhi, India. AIDS Res Hum Retroviruses. 1996;12:1199–202.
131. Lallemant M, Le Coeur S, Samba L, Cheynier D, M'Pelé P, Nzingoula S, Essex M. Mother-to-child transmission of HIV-1 in Congo, central Africa. Congolese Research Group on Mother-to-Child Transmission of HIV. AIDS. 1994;8:1451–6.
132. Lallemant M, Baillou A, Lallemant-Le Coeur S, Nzingoula S, Mampaka M, M'Pelé P, Barin F, Essex M. Maternal antibody response at delivery and perinatal transmission of human immunodeficiency virus type 1 in African women. Lancet. 1994;343:1001–5.
133. Connor EM, Sperling RS, Gelber R, Kiselev P, Scott G, O'Sullivan MJ, VanDyke R, Bey M, Shearer W, et al. Reduction of maternal-infant transmission of human immunodeficiency virus type 1 with zidovudine treatment. Pediatric AIDS Clinical Trials Group Protocol 076 Study Group. N Engl J Med. 1994;331:1173–80.
134. Lurie P, Wolfe SM. Unethical trials of interventions to reduce perinatal transmission of the human immunodeficiency virus in developing countries. N Engl J Med. 1997;337:853–6.
135. Varmus H, Satcher D. Ethical complexities of conducting research in developing countries. N Engl J Med. 1997;337:1003–5.
136. Angell M. The ethics of clinical research in the Third World. N Engl J Med. 1997;337:847–9.

137. Lallemant M, Jourdain G, Le Coeur S, Kim S, Koetsawang S, Comeau AM, Phoolcharoen W, Essex M, McIntosh K, Vithayasai V. A trial of shortened zidovudine regimens to prevent mother-to-child transmission of human immunodeficiency virus type 1. Perinatal HIV Prevention Trial (Thailand) Investigators. N Engl J Med. 2000;343:982–91.
138. Hunt M. Teaming up against AIDS. New York Times Magazine. 2 Mar 1986:Sect. 6:42. https://www.nytimes.com/1986/03/02/magazine/teaming-up-against-aids.html
139. Birx D. Silent invasion: the untold story of the Trump administration, covid-19, and preventing the next pandemic before it's too late. New York: Harper; 2022.
140. Essex M, Mboup S, Kanki PJ, Kalengayi MR, editors. AIDS in Africa. New York: Raven; 1994.
141. Lu Y, Essex M, editors. AIDS in Asia. New York: Kluwer Academic/Plenum Publishers; 2004.
142. DeVita VT Jr, Hellman S, Rosenberg SA, Curran J, Essex M, Fauci AS, editors. AIDS: etiology, diagnosis, treament, and prevention. 4th ed. Philadelphia: J.B. Lippincott; 1997.
143. Ashe A. Days of grace: a memoir. New York: Knopf; 1993.
144. Ndung'u T, Renjifo B, Essex M. Construction and analysis of an infectious human immunodeficiency virus type 1 subtype C molecular clone. J Virol. 2001;75:4964–72. PMCID: PMC114899.
145. Butterfield F. Harvard University: foe of South Africa wins key post on board. New York Times. 6 June 1986:B6.
146. Wachter RM. The fragile coalition: scientists, activists, and AIDS. New York: St. Martin's Press; 1991.
147. Okiror S. Uganda's parliament passes mostly unchanged anti-LGBTQ bill. The Guardian [Internet]. 2 May 2023 [cited 2023 Dec 19]. https://www.theguardian.com/world/2023/may/02/uganda-parliament-passes-anti-lgbtq-bill
148. Essex M. US policy threatens Boston AIDS meeting. Health: A Weekly Journal of Medicine, Science and Society. 23 July 1991:6.
149. Essex M. Sound policy, not AIDS hysteria. AIDS Res Hum Retroviruses. 1991;7:v.
150. Paton E. One of the world's greatest shoppers prepares to share her treasures. New York Times [Internet]. 11 Dec 2023 [cited 2024 Feb 13]. https://www.nytimes.com/2023/11/15/style/mouna-ayoub-chanel-auction.html

151. Masire K. Very brave or very foolish?: memoirs of an African democrat. Lewis SR, editor. Gaborone (BW): Macmillan Botswana; 2006.
152. Novitsky VA, Montano MA, McLane MF, Renjifo B, Vannberg F, Foley BT, Ndung'u TP, Rahman M, Makhema MJ, Marlink R, Essex M. Molecular cloning and phylogenetic analysis of human immunodeficiency virus type 1 subtype C: a set of 23 full-length clones from Botswana. J Virol. 1999;73:4427–32. PMCID: PMC104223.
153. Essex M, Mboup S. Regional variations in the epidemic. In: Essex M, Mboup S, Kanki PJ, Marlink RG, Tlou SD, editors. AIDS in Africa. 2nd ed. New York: Kluwer Academic Plenum Publishers; 2002. p. 1–10.
154. Bbosa N, Kaleebu P, Ssemwanga D. HIV subtype diversity worldwide. Curr Opin HIV AIDS. 2019;14:153–60.
155. Stanecki KA, Walker N. Current estimates and projections for the epidemic. In: Essex M, Mboup S, Kanki PJ, Marlink RG, Tlou SD, editors. AIDS in Africa. 2nd ed. New York: Kluwer Academic Plenum Publishers; 2002. p. 281–296.
156. McCall Smith A. The Saturday big tent wedding party. London: Little, Brown; 2011.
157. United Nations Security Council. Security Council holds debate on impact of AIDS on peace and security in Africa. Press release SC/6781, 10 January 2000. New York: United Nations; 2000.
158. Novitsky V, Rybak N, McLane MF, Gilbert P, Chigwedere P, Klein I, Gaolekwe S, Chang SY, Peter T, Thior I, et al. Identification of human immunodeficiency virus type 1 subtype C Gag-, Tat-, Rev-, and Nef-specific elispot-based cytotoxic T-lymphocyte responses for AIDS vaccine design. J Virol. 2001;75:9210–28. PMCID: PMC114489.
159. Suphaphiphat P, Essex M, Lee TH. Mutations in the V3 stem versus the V3 crown and C4 region have different effects on the binding and fusion steps of human immunodeficiency virus type 1 gp120 interaction with the CCR5 coreceptor. Virology. 2007;360:182–90. PMCID: PMC2014721.
160. Cao H, Agrawal D, Kushner N, Touzjian N, Essex M, Lu Y. Delivery of exogenous protein antigens to major histocompatibility complex class I pathway in cytosol. J Infect Dis. 2002;185:244–51.
161. Fawzi W, Msamanga G, Renjifo B, Spiegelman D, Urassa E, Hashemi L, Antelman G, Essex M, Hunter D. Predictors of intrauterine and intrapartum transmission of HIV-1 among Tanzanian women. AIDS. 2001;15:1157–65.
162. Fawzi W, Msamanga G, Spiegelman D, Renjifo B, Bang H, Kapiga S, Coley J, Hertzmark E, Essex M, Hunter D. Transmission of HIV-1

through breastfeeding among women in Dar es Salaam, Tanzania. J Acquir Immune Defic Syndr. 2002;31:331–8.

163. Renjifo B, Chung M, Gilbert P, Mwakagile D, Msamanga G, Fawzi W, Essex M. In-utero transmission of quasispecies among human immunodeficiency virus type 1 genotypes. Virology. 2003;307:278–82.

164. Makhema J, Wirth KE, Pretorius Holme M, Gaolathe T, Mmalane M, Kadima E, Chakalisa U, Bennett K, Leidner J, Manyake K, et al. Universal testing, expanded treatment, and incidence of HIV infection in Botswana. N Engl J Med. 2019;381:230–42. PMCID: PMC6800102.

165. Essex M, Makhema J, Lockman S. Reaching 90-90-90 in Botswana. Curr Opin HIV AIDS. 2019;14:442–8.

166. Novitsky V, Smith UR, Gilbert P, McLane MF, Chigwedere P, Williamson C, Ndung'u T, Klein I, Chang SY, Peter T, et al. Human immunodeficiency virus type 1 subtype C molecular phylogeny: consensus sequence for an AIDS vaccine design? J Virol. 2002;76:5435–51. PMCID: PMC137027.

167. Doualla-Bell F, Gaseitsiwe S, Ndungú T, Modukanele M, Peter T, Novitsky V, Ndwapi N, Tendani G, Avalos A, Wester W, et al. Mutations and polymorphisms associated with antiretroviral drugs in HIV-1C-infected African patients. Antivir Chem Chemother. 2004;15:189–200.

168. Bussmann C, Rotz P, Ndwapi N, Baxter D, Bussmann H, Wester CW, Ncube P, Avalos A, Mine M, Mabe E, et al. Strengthening healthcare capacity through a responsive, country-specific, training standard: the KITSO AIDS training program's support of Botswana's national antiretroviral therapy rollout. Open AIDS J. 2008;2:10–6. PMCID: PMC2556202.

169. Bussmann H, Wester CW, Ndwapi N, Grundmann N, Gaolathe T, Puvimanasinghe J, Avalos A, Mine M, Seipone K, Essex M, Degruttola V, Marlink RG. Five-year outcomes of initial patients treated in Botswana's National Antiretroviral Treatment Program. AIDS. 2008;22:2303–11. PMCID: PMC2853026.

170. Lockman S, Shapiro RL, Smeaton LM, Wester C, Thior I, Stevens L, Chand F, Makhema J, Moffat C, Asmelash A, et al. Response to antiretroviral therapy after a single, peripartum dose of nevirapine. N Engl J Med. 2007;356:135–47.

171. Cohen MS, Chen YQ, McCauley M, Gamble T, Hosseinipour MC, Kumarasamy N, Hakim JG, Kumwenda J, Grinsztejn B, Pilotto JHS, et al. Antiretroviral therapy for the prevention of HIV-1 transmission. N Engl J Med. 2016;375:830–9. PMCID: PMC5049503.

172. Novitsky V, Ndung'u T, Wang R, Bussmann H, Chonco F, Makhema J, De Gruttola V, Walker BD, Essex M. Extended high viremics: a substantial fraction of individuals maintain high plasma viral RNA levels after acute HIV-1 subtype C infection. AIDS. 2011;25:1515–22. PMCID: PMC3544358.
173. Novitsky V, Kuhnert D, Moyo S, Widenfelt E, Okui L, Essex M. Phylodynamic analysis of HIV sub-epidemics in Mochudi, Botswana. Epidemics. 2015;13:44–55. PMCID: PMC4664890.
174. Gaolathe T, Wirth KE, Holme MP, Makhema J, Moyo S, Chakalisa U, Yankinda EK, Lei Q, Mmalane M, Novitsky V, et al. Botswana's progress toward achieving the 2020 UNAIDS 90-90-90 antiretroviral therapy and virological suppression goals: a population-based survey. Lancet HIV. 2016;3:e221–30. PMCID: PMC5146754.
175. Magosi LE, Tchetgen ET, Novitsky V, Pretorius Holme M, Moore J, Bachanas P, Lebelonyane R, Fraser C, Moyo S, Hurwitz KE, et al. Unpacking sources of transmission in HIV prevention trials with deep-sequence pathogen data. Nat Commun. 2026;17(1):3935. PMCID: PMC13128811.
176. UNAIDS. 90-90-90: an ambitious treatment target to help end the AIDS epidemic. Geneva: Joint United Nations Programme on HIV/AIDS (UNAIDS). 2014.
177. GBD 2021 HIV Collaborators. Global, regional, and national burden of HIV/AIDS, 1990–2021, and forecasts to 2050, for 204 countries and territories: the Global Burden of Disease Study 2021. Lancet HIV. 2024;11:e807–22. PMCID: PMC11612058.
178. Wang R, Wang J, Hu T, Zhou X-H. Population-level effectiveness of COVID-19 vaccination program in the United States: causal analysis based on structural nested mean model. Vaccines (Basel). 2022;10. PMCID: PMC9144931.
179. Institute of Medicine. Assessment of future scientific needs for live variola virus. Washington: National Academies Press; 1999.
180. Noack R. After long banning polio campaigns, Taliban declares war on the disease. Washington Post [Internet]. 5 Dec 2023 [cited 2024 Mar 1]. https://www.washingtonpost.com/world/2023/12/05/taliban-afghanistan-polio-vaccination/
181. Sun LH, Weber L. Florida surgeon general defies science amid measles outbreak. Washington Post [Internet]. 22 Feb 2024 [cited 2024 Mar 1]. https://www.washingtonpost.com/health/2024/02/22/florida-measles-outbreak-ladapo/

182. Covid Crisis Group. Lessons from the COVID war: an investigative report. New York: PublicAffairs; 2023.
183. Krieger N, Testa C, Chen JT, Hanage WP, McGregor AJ. Relationship of political ideology of US federal and state elected officials and key COVID pandemic outcomes following vaccine rollout to adults: April 2021–March 2022. Lancet Reg Health Am. 2022;16:100384. PMCID: PMC9621695.
184. Weber L. How the anti-vaccine movement is gaining power in statehouses. Washington Post [Internet]. 21 Feb 2024 [cited 2024 Mar 1]. https://www.washingtonpost.com/health/2023/12/22/anti-vaccine-covid/
185. Cutler DM, Summers LH. The COVID-19 pandemic and the $16 trillion virus. JAMA. 2020;324:1495–6. PMCID: PMC7604733.
186. Lupica M. Robert B. Parker's fallout. New York: G.P. Putnam's Sons; 2022.
187. McGraw M, Stein S. It's been exactly one year since Trump suggested injecting bleach. We've never been the same. Politico [Internet]. 23 Apr 2021 [cited 2025 Aug 2]. Available from: https://www.politico.com/news/2021/04/23/trump-bleach-one-year-484399
188. Frum D. Why the COVID deniers won. Atlantic Monthly [Internet]. February 2025 [cited 2025 Aug 2]. https://www.theatlantic.com/magazine/archive/2025/03/covid-deniers-anti-vax-public-health-politics-polarization/681435/
189. Stolberg SG. Trump withdraws U.S. from World Health Organization. New York Times [Internet]. 20 Jan 2025 [cited 2025 Oct 21]. Available from: https://www.nytimes.com/2025/01/20/us/politics/trump-world-health-organization.html
190. Mandavilli A. The C.D.C.'s vaccine meeting: what to watch for. New York Times [Internet]. 25 Jun 2025 [cited 2025 Oct 21]. Available from: https://www.nytimes.com/2025/06/25/health/acip-cdc-vaccines-kennedy.html
191. Sun LH, Weber L. How vaccine critics appointed by RFK Jr. could limit access to shots. Washington Post [Internet]. 13 Jun 2025 [cited 2025 Oct 21]. Available from: https://www.washingtonpost.com/health/2025/06/13/rfk-jr-vaccine-committee-overhaul/
192. Masih N, Westfall S. RFK Jr. says U.S. will stop funding global vaccine alliance Gavi. Washington Post [Internet]. 26 June 2025 [cited 2025 Oct 21]. Available from: https://www.washingtonpost.com/health/2025/06/26/rfk-jr-vaccine-gavi-funding-cut/

193. Stone W. RFK Jr.'s vaccine policy sparks a lawsuit from the American Academy of Pediatrics. NPR [Internet]. 8 July 2025 [cited 2025 Oct 21]. Available from: https://www.npr.org/transcripts/nx-s1-5459978
194. Mandavilli A. Kennedy scales back the number of vaccines recommended for children. New York Times [Internet]. 5 Jan 2026 [cited 2026 Jan 23]. Available from: https://www.nytimes.com/2026/01/05/health/children-vaccines-cdc-kennedy.html
195. Sun LH. U.S. measles cases reach 33-year high as outbreaks spread. Washington Post [Internet]. 7 June 2025 [cited 2025 Oct 21]. Available from: https://www.washingtonpost.com/health/2025/07/07/measles-cases-hit-record/
196. Rosenbluth T. Measles cases spike in South Carolina. New York Times [Internet]. 9 Jan 2026 [cited 2026 Jan 23]. Available from: https://www.nytimes.com/2026/01/09/well/measles-outbreak-new-cases-south-carolina.html
197. Westfall S, Sun LH. Global health experts sound alarm over RFK Jr., citing Samoa outbreak. Washington Post [Internet]. 16 Nov 2024 [cited 2025 Oct 21]. Available from: https://www.washingtonpost.com/world/2024/11/15/rfk-jr-global-health-samoa-kennedy/
198. Williamson E. Hawaii governor, a doctor, blames Kennedy for measles deaths in Samoa. New York Times [Internet]. 28 Jan 2025 [cited 2025 Oct 21]. Available from: https://www.nytimes.com/2025/01/28/us/politics/measles-rfk-jr.html
199. Frances A. Autism rates have increased 60-fold. I played a role in that. New York Times [Internet]. 23 June 2025 [cited 2025 Oct 21]. Available from: https://www.nytimes.com/2025/06/23/opinion/why-autism-rates-increased.html
200. McNeil DG Jr. RFK Jr.'s view of autism is wrong – but profitable. Washington Post [Internet]. 1 May 2025 [cited 2025 Oct 21]. Available from: https://www.washingtonpost.com/opinions/2025/05/01/rfk-autism-study-science/
201. Tsouderos T. "Miracle drug" called junk science. Chicago Tribune [Internet]. 19 August 2019 [cited 2025 Oct 21]. Available from: https://www.chicagotribune.com/2009/05/21/miracle-drug-called-junk-science-2/
202. Wakefield AJ, Murch SH, Anthony A, Linnell J, Casson DM, Malik M, Berelowitz M, Dhillon AP, Thomson MA, Harvey P, Valentine A, Davies SE, Walker-Smith JA. Ileal-lymphoid-nodular hyperplasia,

non-specific colitis, and pervasive developmental disorder in children. Lancet. 1998;351:637–41.

203. Deer B. The doctor who fooled the world: science, deception, and the war on vaccines. Baltimore (MD): Johns Hopkins University Press; 2020.
204. Hooper E. The river: a journey to the source of HIV and AIDS. Boston (MA): Little, Brown and Co.; 1999.
205. Koprowski H. AIDS and the polio vaccine. Science. 1992;257:1024, 1026–7.
206. Jha HK. Canceling Moderna's bird flu contract could be Robert Kennedy's most reckless act yet. Boston Globe [Internet]. 3 Jun 2025 [cited 2025 Oct 21]. Available from: https://www.bostonglobe.com/2025/06/03/opinion/robert-kennedy-jr-moderna-vaccine-cancellation-contract/
207. Sweeney E. Trump slams "totally FALSE" claim he was snubbed by Harvard: "I never applied." Boston Globe [Internet]. 3 Jun 2025 [cited 2025 Oct 21]. Available from: https://www.bostonglobe.com/2025/06/03/metro/trump-refutes-claim-harvard-michael-wolff/
208. Commander A. Donald Trump shoots down rumor he applied to Harvard. Newsweek [Internet]. 2 Jun 2025 [cited 2025 Oct 21]. Available from: https://www.newsweek.com/donald-trump-shoots-down-rumor-he-applied-harvard-2080095
209. Arsenault M, Ryan A, Leung S. Trump once swore revenge on the Pritzker family. Decades later, Penny Pritzker is helping lead Harvard's resistance against him. Boston Globe [Internet]. 22 May 2025 [cited 2025 Oct 21]. Available from: https://www.bostonglobe.com/2025/05/22/business/penny-pritzker-harvard-trump-resistance/
210. Damiano M, Burns H. Trump vs. Harvard fight gets personal: White House wants Garber out as school girds for long slog, changes. Boston Globe. 1 Jun 2025:A1.
211. Bruni F, Douthat R, Summers LH. "Are we past peak Harvard?": 3 writers mull higher education's woes: round table. New York Times [Internet]. 22 Jun 2025 [cited 2025 Oct 21]. Available from: https://www.nytimes.com/2025/06/22/opinion/trump-higher-education-harvard.html
212. Fares M, Cherelus G. Trump loves "the poorly educated" ... and social media clamors. Reuters [Internet]. 24 Feb 2016 [cited 2025 Oct 29]. Available from: https://www.reuters.com/article/world/trump-loves-the-poorly-educated-and-social-media-clamors-idUSKCN0VX2DE/

213. Pasquini N. How MAGA went mainstream at Harvard: Trump, TikTok, and the pandemic are reshaping Gen Z politics. Harvard Magazine [Internet]. 8 Aug 2025 [cited 2025 Oct 21]. Available from: https://www.harvardmagazine.com/students/harvard-young-americans-conservative-turn
214. Damiano M, Burns H. Trump administration says Harvard funding cuts are punishment for "race discrimination." Boston Globe [Internet]. 28 May 2025 [cited 2025 Oct 29]. Available from: https://www.bostonglobe.com/2025/05/27/metro/trump-harvard-funding-contracts-cuts/
215. Schmidt MS, Bender MC. Trump administration says it is halting Harvard's ability to enroll international students. New York Times [Internet]. 29 May 2025 [cited 2025 Oct 29]. Available from: https://www.nytimes.com/2025/05/22/us/politics/trump-harvard-international-students.html
216. McDaniel J, Svrluga S. Trump vs. Harvard: a timeline of how the fight escalated. Washington Post [Internet]. 3 Sep 2025 [cited 2025 Oct 21]. Available from: https://www.washingtonpost.com/education/interactive/2025/timeline-trump-harvard/
217. Perez J Jr. Trump threatens Harvard patents worth hundreds of millions. Politico [Internet]. 8 Aug 2025 [cited 2025 Oct 29]. Available from: https://www.politico.com/news/2025/08/08/trump-harvard-patents-00500814
218. Blinder A, Bender MC. Trump administration renews attacks on Harvard with negotiations uncertain. New York Times [Internet]. 9 Jul 2025 [cited 2025 Oct 30]. Available from: https://www.nytimes.com/2025/07/09/us/politics/trump-harvard-data-accreditation.html
219. Wosen J. Judge issues preliminary injunction blocking Trump cuts to NIH research overhead payments. STAT News [Internet]. 5 Mar 2025 [cited 2025 Oct 30]. Available from: https://www.statnews.com/2025/03/05/nih-indirect-costs-lawsuit-federal-judge-extends-order-blocking-trump-cuts/
220. Mueller B. Trump administration slashes research into L.G.B.T.Q. health. New York Times [Internet]. 4 May 2025 [cited 2025 Oct 30]. Available from: https://www.nytimes.com/2025/05/04/health/trump-administration-slashes-research-into-lgbtq-health.html
221. Stein R. Public health experts dismayed by RFK Jr.'s defunding of mRNA vaccine research. NPR [Internet]. 6 Aug 2025 [cited 2025 Oct 30]. Available from: https://www.npr.org/sections/shots-health-news/2025/08/06/nx-s1-5493544/rfk-defunding-mrna-vaccine-research

222. Willett WC, Green A, Stampfer MJ, Speizer FE, Colditz GA, Rosner B, Monson RR, Stason W, Hennekens CH. Relative and absolute excess risks of coronary heart disease among women who smoke cigarettes. N Engl J Med. 1987;317:1303–9.
223. Ignatius D. This is what a war on knowledge looks like. Washington Post [Internet]. 3 Jun 2025 [cited 2025 Oct 21]. Available from: https://www.washingtonpost.com/opinions/2025/06/03/maga-science-advantage-destruction-mao/
224. Nature Index. Institution rankings [Internet]. 1 Jan 2025 – 31 Dec 2025 [cited 2025 Oct 1]. Available from: https://www.nature.com/nature-index/institution-outputs/generate/all/global/academic
225. Pasquini N. What happens if Harvard loses its international students: research, revenue, and global standing are all on the line. Harvard Magazine [Internet]. 11 Jun 2025 [cited 2025 Oct 21]. Available from: https://www.harvardmagazine.com/2025/06/harvard-trump-international-students
226. Thornton C. Trump is slashing billions from Harvard. Here's a breakdown of the federal funding that's been lost. Boston Globe [Internet]. 28 May 2025 [cited 2025 Oct 21]. Available from: https://www.bostonglobe.com/2025/05/28/metro/how-much-money-has-trump-cut-from-harvard-heres-a-breakdown/
227. Saul S. Judge blocks Trump proclamation barring Harvard's international students. New York Times [Internet]. 25 Jun 2025 [cited 2025 Oct 30]. Available from: https://www.nytimes.com/2025/06/23/us/harvard-trump-international-students.html

Index